Bodymind

The Whole Person Health Book

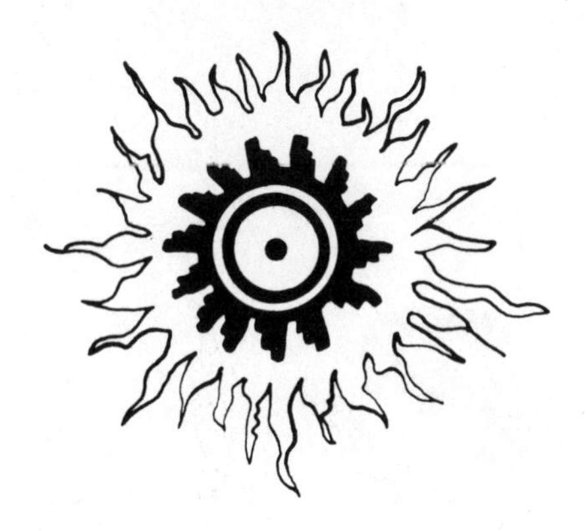

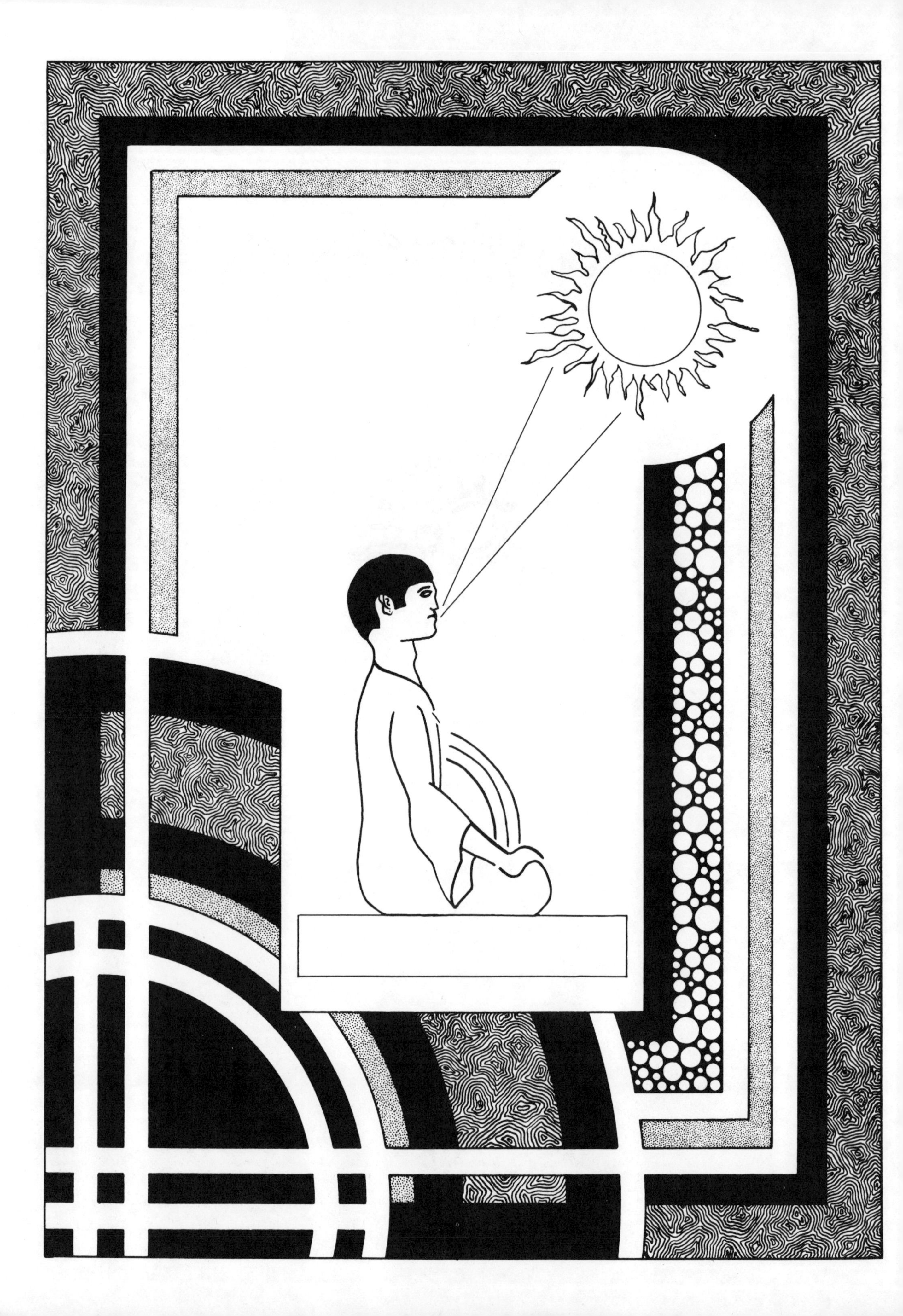

Bodymind

The Whole Person Health Book

by
Don Ethan Miller

illustrated by
Julian Asher Miller

PRENTICE-HALL, INC. Englewood Cliffs, New Jersey

Design by Linda Huber

Unless otherwise indicated, all drawings and photographs by Julian Asher Miller.

Decorations on pages ii, iii, 1, 23, 115, 183, and 201 from *Original Art Deco Designs,* by William Rowe, Dover Publications, Inc.

Bodymind: The Whole Person Health Book, by Don Ethan Miller

Printed in the United States of America
Prentice-Hall International, Inc., London
Prentice-Hall of Australia, Pty. Ltd., North Sydney
Prentice-Hall of Canada, Ltd., Toronto
Prentice-Hall of India Private Ltd., New Delhi
Prentice-Hall of Japan, Inc., Toyko

10 9 8 7 6 5 4 3 2

Library of Congress Cataloging in Publication Data

Miller, Don Ethan.
Bodymind; the whole person health book.
1. Hygiene, Personal. 2. Mental hygiene.
I. Miller, Julian Asher, illus. II. Title.
[DNLM: 1. Health. 2. Hygiene. QT180 M65b 1974]
RA776.5.M5 613 73-20280
ISBN 0-13-079616-6

To Phyllis,
for her cornucopia
of positive reinforcements; and Sigmund,
for his relentless
clear-mindedness:
to my parents, for their love.

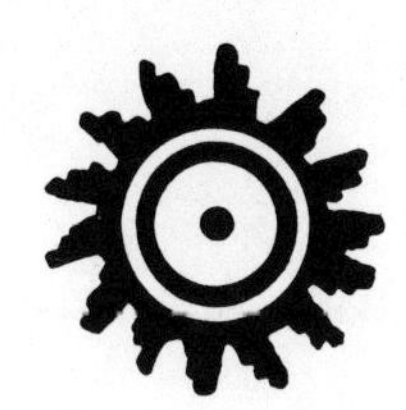

Contents

Love man because you are he.

Love animals and plants because
you were they, and now they follow you like faithful co-workers
and slaves.

Love your body; only with it may
you fight on this earth and
turn matter into spirit.

Love matter. God clings to it
tooth and nail, and fights.
Fight with him.

Die every day. Be born every day.
Deny everything you have every day.
The superior virtue is not to be
free, but to fight for freedom.

Nikos Kazantzakis, *The Saviors of God*

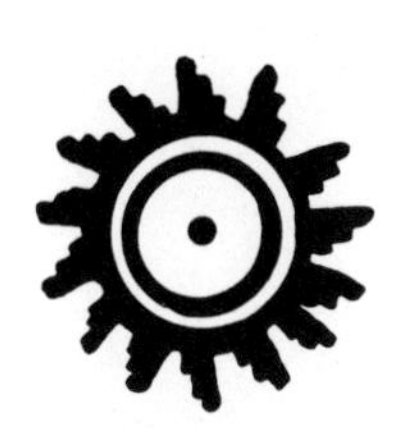

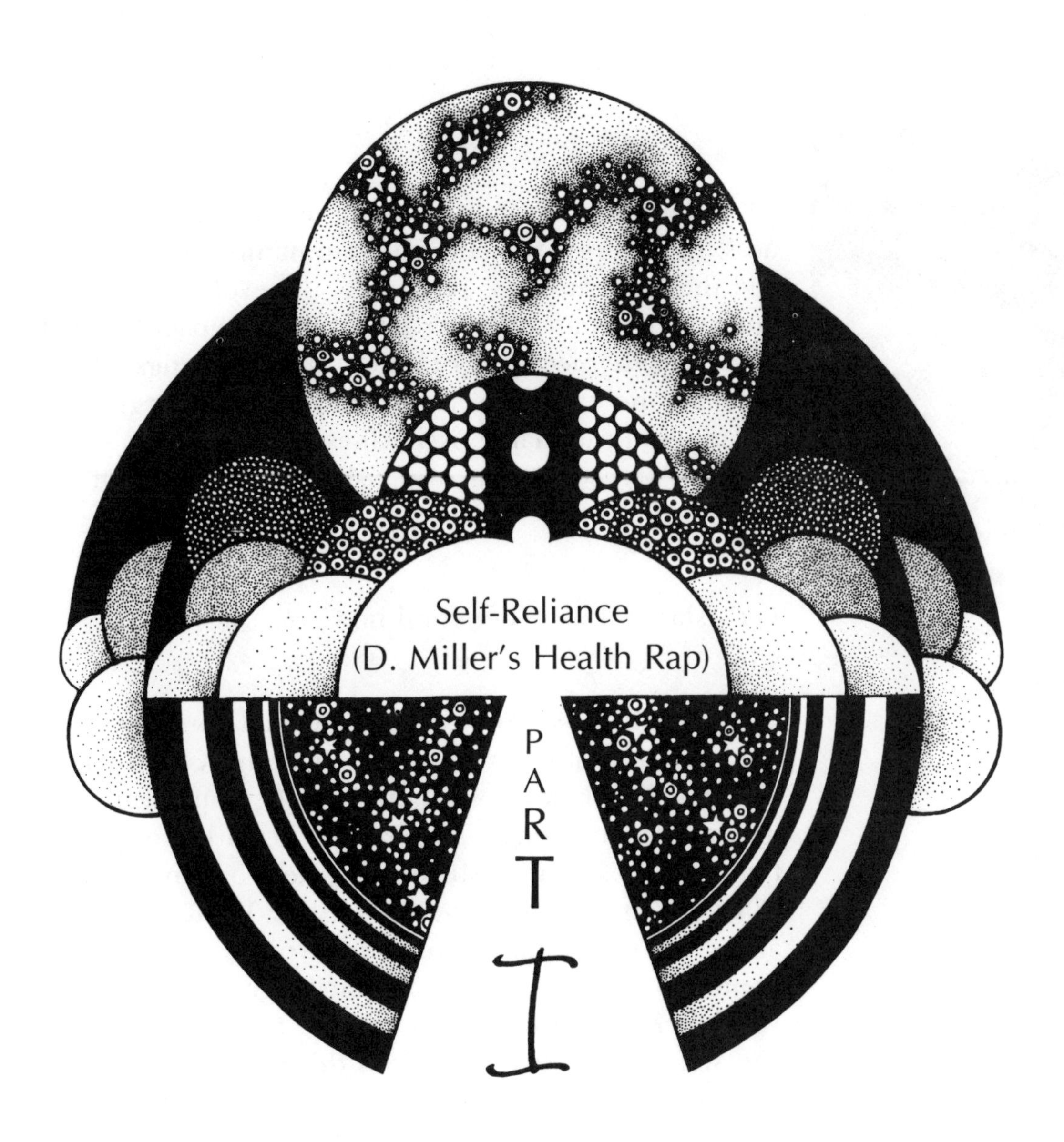
Self-Reliance
(D. Miller's Health Rap)
PART
I

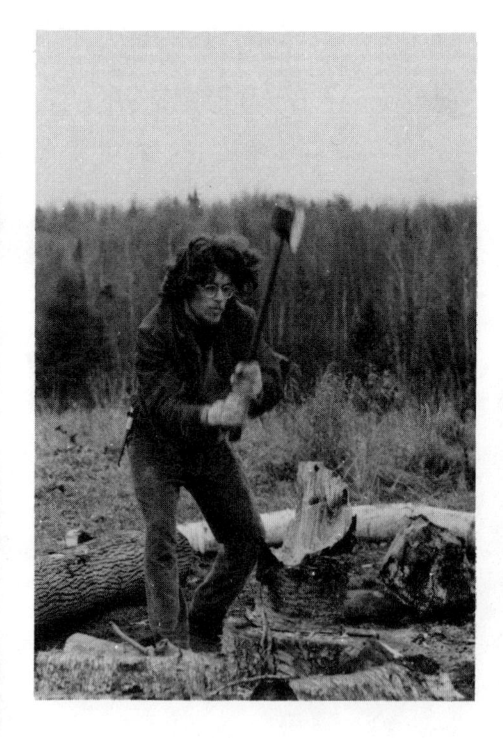

The Chinese have a word for it—
tzu-li keng-sheng—which means
regeneration through one's own effort,
a kind of Emersonian self-reliance.

NEW YORK *Post*, 1972

(D. Miller's Health Rap—being a discussion of awareness, life-energy, the authoritarian nature of our society and the powerlessness of people, the evolution of the human animal and his/her fall from psychosomatic balance, and the necessity of a new life that brings together the unrepressed physical/natural energies and the modern rational consciousness in an organic state of health. Proceed at your own risk. And in your own good time.)

Let's start with the here and now: *How do you feel?*

I mean, how do you *really* feel? Could you describe the condition of every part of your body? Could you report on all muscles, joints, and bones? Your heart and lungs? Your nervous system? The circulation of your blood? How's your posture—slouched, or tensed up? What's your attitude as you read this? What physical and social environment surrounds you, and do you feel good about it? What can you smell right now? What can you hear? What things near you are alive, and how do you sense their life? What does this make you think about? Staying in the present: how do you *feel?*

Are you aware of your whole body-and-mind as one unit, its physical weight concentrated between your hips, at your natural center of gravity? Or are there muscle tensions (shoulders? neck? face?) pulling upwards and making you fight gravity for no useful reason?

Do you have the sensation that your blood, your inner electricity, your life-energy is flowing, evenly and uninterrupted, through your whole bodymind? Or do you feel it concentrated in some places and not reaching other parts at all? For example, do your legs feel deadened, and your eyes overworked? That's from sitting in chairs and car seats too much of the day, everyday. Right now do you have less energy, less *feeling,* in your hips, your pelvis, your buttocks, your genitals than you do in your hands, your eyes, your mouth? Why is that, do you think?

Maybe it's the way you're sitting. Maybe your belly is too full, or too fat, and it hangs over your groin and immobilizes your hips. Maybe the clothes you're wearing restrict the free movement of your waist, your hips, your legs—and you've been accustomed to that imprisonment for so long you don't even notice it.

Where would you say your body's center is? Would you say that more energy is flowing upwards, or downwards, from this place? How often do you *allow* energy to flow downwards, into your thighs, your genitals, your buttocks, your naked feet?

Perhaps you do so, rarely, fleetingly, even reluctantly —when you run for a bus, or climb a few flights of stairs, or in the all too brief minutes you give to making love. But is it enough? Do you feel balanced, centered, unified? How does it feel to have *your* body, to be *in* your body, to *be* your body?

What about your thoughts? Your dreams? Your deepest feelings? Do your strongest emotions stay locked inside you, so that you don't even know them yourself, except as a kind of jailor maintaining "order" above all else? When was the last time you sang just for the pleasure of it?

Do you ever shout at the top of your lungs because you *want* to? How do you like your job? Your home life? Do you feel you really know what's going on, in your own life and in the rest of the world you live in? Or do you just try to "get by" and forget the rest? What do you do in situations you are afraid of, or with people you are afraid of? What things *are* you afraid of?

And what, after all, are you doing being *alive* on this strange and beautiful planet? What has your life been like up to now? It doesn't matter if you're 16, or 35, or 86—answer this question: Where would you like to go from here? It's up to you!

Come on and walk with me awhile. I can show you some interesting places and we'll talk about some things. What do you *think* about all day long? When did you last walk barefoot on soft pine needles? How do you really *feel?*

To make any lasting improvement in your life, even if it's something relatively simple like losing weight or giving up cigarettes, you have to step outside your normal way of doing things. You have to give up your everyday reality for a while and look closely at yourself. This is something no one else can do for you.

Even the most complete medical examination or the most candid psychiatric interview will not reveal one-tenth of the things that you already know about yourself! All too often these days, stories like this take place in real life: A man walks into the doctor's office, requesting an electrocardiogram because he fears his heart is failing. The doctor examines him and finds him perfectly normal. The machine tests him and detects no sign of heart trouble. He leaves the office. The next day he has a heart attack and dies.

In some way the man *knew* what the doctor and the machine could not know. The messages from his own body, which he had been ignoring for a long time, finally got through, and he heard them. If he had heard sooner, he might have lived.

All the information you need is already there within you. You just have to rediscover and release this knowledge, to use it. But how? As a first step, get rid of all those anti-self ideas about the experts, the established authorities, the accepted methods, the modern machinery. Free yourself of all those preconceptions that prevent you from hearing your own voice, and heeding the messages of your own bodymind. "Health is the truth of the body." The cure resides in you.

They say truth is a pathless land. It is the same for true health—total, mind-and-body health: there are no broad, well-paved, easily followed roads to get you there. Real health *is* attainable by everyone—but not in the same way for each person. It's an individual affair. There is no single way that can be followed successfully by all people.

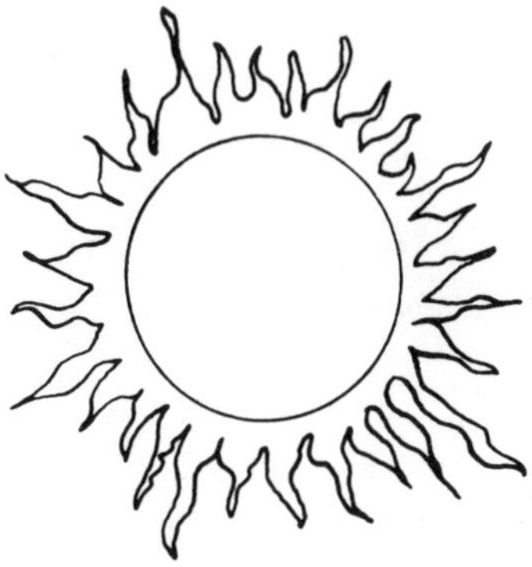

> Discard all theologies and all belief . . . the whole principle that someone else knows and you do not know, that the one who knows is going to teach you.
>
> KRISHNAMURTI

I'm not here to *teach* you. I don't want you to eat what I eat, practice what I practice, or live the way I live. Almost everything I know, I taught myself, and I'm not interested in becoming anyone's guru! But what I *can* do is show you some ways of teaching *yourself.* You can become healthier, you can live with more energy, more passion, more intensity. You can live less under the rule of fear and more in the fresh air of confidence and love. You can take your life into your own hands and make of it what you will. (But not if you put it into mine!)

I cannot tell you when to breathe, how deeply to

breathe, how quickly or how slowly to breathe. I *can* tell you of the changes I experience as I alter my breathing —changes of body, emotions, and mind. I can tell you how the Aikido master practices breathing, and how the Yogi does. I can tell you about oxygen consumption, tidal volume, and training effect. I can do everything possible to make you *aware* of your own shallow breathing, and aware of the possibility of a deeper, more natural, and infinitely healthier breathing pattern. But I cannot teach you to breathe!

In our society it seems that everything is done by someone else. You need food: you buy vegetables someone else has grown, eat meat someone else has killed, chew bread someone else has baked. You need shelter: so you sleep in a house someone else has built, sit in chairs someone else has fashioned, eat from a bowl you did not carve, wear clothes you did not weave. You drive a car whose design you could never have imagined, made from metals you did not mine, running on gas you did not pump and oil you did not drain from the earth, with tires from rubber trees you did not tap.

I'm not saying we should immediately dismantle the machinery of civilization and return to the old ways. It's too late for that. There are too many of us and, most importantly, it's not the civilization itself that is the real problem, but the insidious state of mind behind it. This *idea* we have that we cannot do anything for ourselves; that there are others who can certainly do it better, if we only have enough money to pay them. The idea that "someone else knows." This is the real problem, this deep-seated sense of powerlessness that carries over to every area of our lives, invades and distorts even our most basic human feelings and life processes.

Several years ago in New York City a woman was attacked, chased, stabbed, and finally murdered—while 50 or 60 people watched from their windows and did nothing. Why? Because in their minds they had assigned the function of helping people in distress and fighting crime to *someone else*—the police. Their natural instincts must have been to help, to do *something* to prevent the murder unfolding on the sidewalk below. But no, the mentality was ingrained in them which said: It's not your business, there are special people who take care of these things, don't involve yourself. . . .

The same thing happens in the political sphere. The "leaders" are supposed to know; we're supposed to follow. Even in the various forms of opposition to the government, it's the same thing—leaders who know, followers who don't know. Do we really take part in shaping the world with our individual votes, our ignored signatures on letters of petition or protest, our membership in one organization or another? Is the world in such good shape that we should go on accepting that those we allow to lead us really do "know"?

I am not saying we should now do away with the police, refrain from voting, abolish the government. It seems that at the present we cannot do without these things—because of the way we are. But the way we are is not so good. We have evil, senseless wars that destroy millions, public works that do not work, promises that are not kept, the natural environment destroyed to build cities not fit to live in—and taxes we must pay to keep the whole thing going. Inevitably, in each of us there grows the conviction that everything is beyond our control.

We are taught and conditioned from an early age not to trust ourselves. Not to rely on our own experiences, perceptions, or feelings about anything. Even about our bodies and the way they feel. Even about our minds. Good health becomes, not your own personal love affair with life, but the property and province of the health specialists, "those who know" about such things.

If you feel bad, they say take a pill, have a drink, sit down and watch television, wait for the doctor, go see a psychiatrist, a priest, a guru, someone who knows. If you need a bigger change, they say go on a vacation, take up a hobby, go on this diet, follow this system or that method or this exercise program, the way of someone who knows. Don't try to be your own mechanic, your own lawyer, your own psychiatrist, your own carpenter or food producer or spiritual adviser—and certainly not your own doctor. For God's sake don't try to heal yourself, don't dare to figure things out for yourself; the whole house of cards might collapse if you did!

But even a willing follower gets into trouble. All the people who are supposed to know say different things! Some authorities tell you to eat only grains and vegetables; some say eat only fruit. Some say you need a "balanced" diet including animal protein, fruits, vegetables, and dairy products. Some say you've got to supplement *any* diet with vitamin pills, mineral tablets, brewer's yeast, and a million other things. And then there were the Plains tribes of American Indians who lived and enjoyed tremendous health and vitality—on a diet of four pounds of buffalo meat per day!

Some health "experts" will tell you that health depends entirely on your body chemistry, on the presence or absence of certain essential nutrients (proteins, vitamins, minerals, trace elements). Others say you will become healthy by performing certain slow, gentle exercises every day. Still others insist you must exert yourself strenuously, make yourself sweat every day. Some talk of illnesses and disorders as psychosomatic ("psyche" = mind, "soma" = body), and of the necessity of strengthening your will to live. Still others deal with spiritual matters and propose meditation, prayer, or religious faith as the only true path to health.

There is some truth in all these ways. And some falsehood. Many of them actually do succeed in restoring some people to physical health and emotional well-being. The problem is that in following one system you are supposed to accept it as right, and all the others as wrong. Worse, you are also asked to deny the validity of your own feelings, perceptions, and instinctual wisdom.

For example: You're on a "macrobiotic" diet, eating brown rice and vegetables. You get a slight cold. Your body needs Vitamin C to resist the infection. It communicates this need to your brain, where it takes the form of a craving for wild blackberries or fresh-squeezed orange juice. But citrus and other fruits are not allowed on the macrobiotic diet, which you believe in wholeheartedly. Do you heed your body's message and eat fruit, or do you follow the System, rejecting your own psychosomatic information as being less valuable than the theories of those in the know?

It's clear to me. At exactly such points we've got to say *no* to "those who know" and *yes* to ourselves. *We must begin to become self-reliant.*

That "no," and that "yes," may be of greater importance than we realize. Starting with our own bodies, and our own minds, we can reclaim them and make them truly our own. This self-reliance grows and carries over into other areas—our work, our social relations, our whole lives. It may even begin to turn around the whole nature of our unhealthy civilization. People who trust themselves, who know themselves and follow no one, also trust others, understand others, do not wish for power over others. Starting with ourselves, we can remake the world.

Without health and self-reliance, our lives go off in strange directions; we can be made to do anything. But we have the choice of being free and independent creatures, we have the right and the capacity to become strong, and beautiful, and kind. These are not just words, they are real human possibilities. You can make them real.

We all feel that life was simpler long ago, when man lived in harmony with nature and followed his own instincts. When he didn't *think* so much—and didn't have to. When thinking and feeling were not enemies, work and pleasure were not opposites, the mind and the body were not divided. When there were no cities, no nations, no kings, no presidents, no wars, no money, no jails, no cars, no machines. Maybe such a time never existed. Maybe it did.

We do know that man's brain continued to develop long after his body reached its present form. Human beings 40,000 years ago were physically the same as we are. Actually, their brain *size* was the same too. The difference is the amount of energy that goes up to the forebrain, the cerebral cortex—the seat of the conscious mind.

In "civilized" man the conscious mind dominates existence. Thinking supersedes the emotions, the instincts, and almost all the messages of the body. As man learns, new nerve patterns become imprinted and recorded in the forebrain. In the course of human evolution this "new" brain has become the locus of more energy—in the form of electrical charges following these new patterns. Meanwhile, the "old" brain, the primitive rear brain (cerebellum) and midbrain and spinal cord, along with the rest of the body, have remained the same during this development, if in fact they have not declined in energy. In short, our mental evolution has made us top-heavy.

In some way man has felt this imbalance for a long time. We have tremendous knowledge about *things,* we have vast technologies that can put men on the moon, prevent diseases of all kinds, destroy whole populations with the press of a button. Yet who among us *feels as alive* as the cat does, or the eagle, or the dolphin? In the Biblical sense we have eaten from the Tree of Knowledge, but not from the Tree of Life.

In the millennia of struggle, through all the terrors of

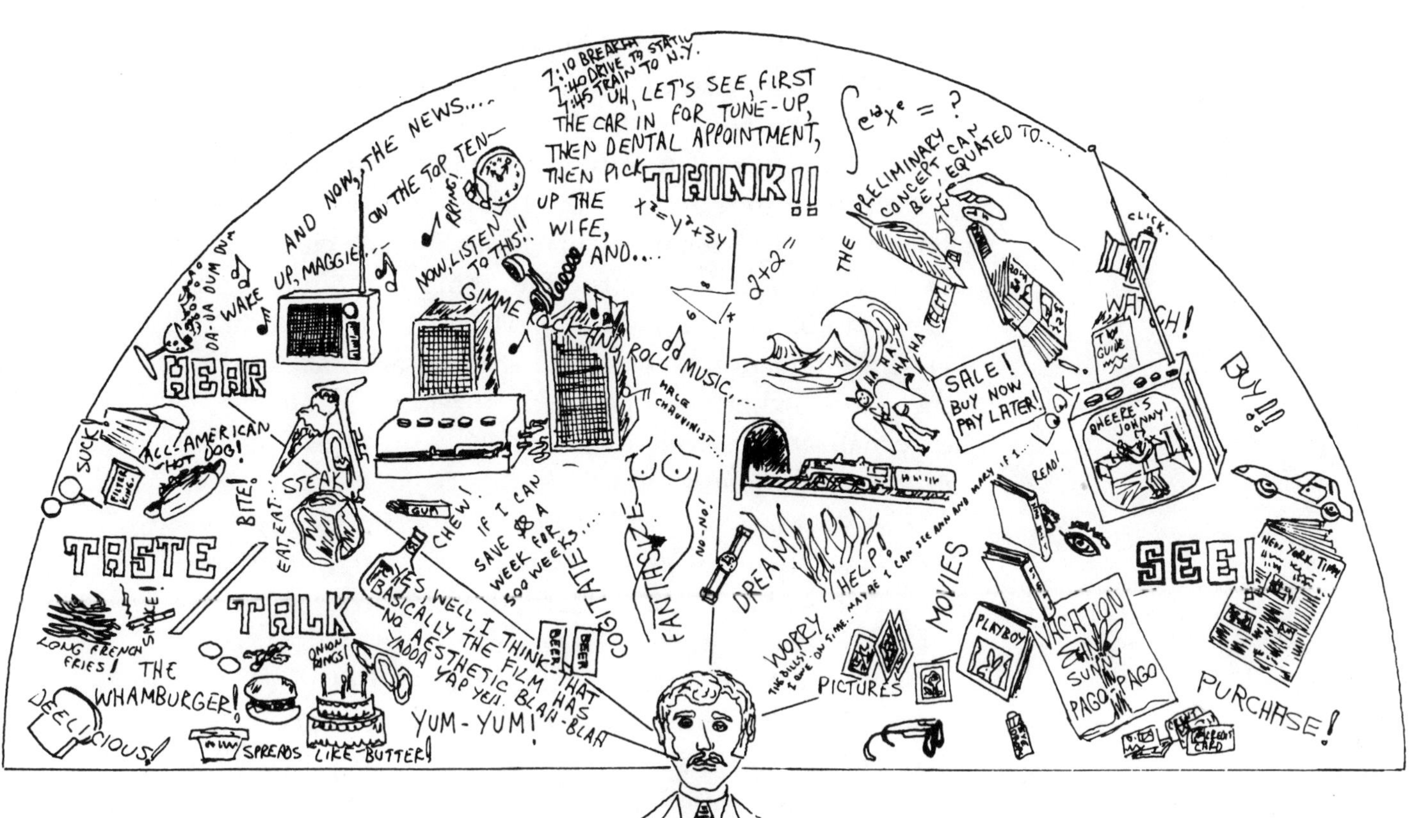

HEAR
DA-DA DUM DUM
WAKE UP, MAGGIE...
AND NOW, THE NEWS....
ON THE TOP TEN—
RING!
NOW, LISTEN TO THIS!!
GIMME ROCK AND ROLL MUSIC...
UH, LET'S SEE, FIRST THE CAR IN FOR TUNE-UP, THEN DENTAL APPOINTMENT, THEN PICK UP THE WIFE, AND....
THINK!!
$x^2=y^2+3y$
2+2=
THE PRELIMINARY CONCEPT CAN BE EQUATED TO....
CLICK
WATCH!
TV GUIDE
SALE! BUY NOW PAY LATER!
HA HA HA HA
LOOK!
WHEERE'S JOHNNY!
BUY!!!
READ!
SEE!
NEW YORK TIMES
SUCK!
ALL-AMERICAN HOT DOG!
STEAK
BITE!
EAT, EAT
GUM
CHEW!
TASTE
TALK
SMOKE!
LONG FRENCH FRIES!
THE WHAMBURGER!
DEELICIOUS!
SPREADS LIKE BUTTER!
ONION RINGS!
YUM-YUM!
YES, WELL, I THINK THAT BASICALLY THE FILM HAS NO AESTHETIC YADDA YAP YEH. BLAH-BLAH
BEER
IF I CAN SAVE $5 A WEEK FOR 500 WEEKS....
COGITATE
MALE CHAUVINIST...
FANTASIZE
NO-NO!
DREAM
HELP!
WORRY
MOVIES
PICTURES
PLAYBOY
VACATION
SUNNY PAGO-PAGO
PURCHASE!

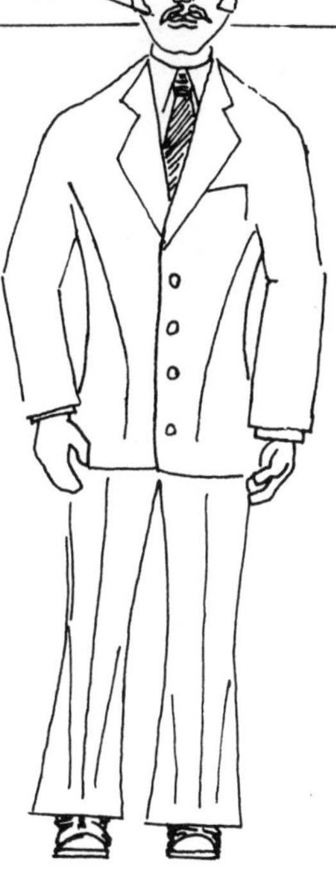

our history, in joy and in sorrow, man has been seeking to restore the balance, to regain the life we have somehow lost. We have evolved in these 40,000 years, but our growth has been only of the mind. The energy of our evolving has gone to the brain only, which rules us now; we build ever more machines, bigger cities, greater weapons of destruction, more complicated structures of abstract thought. Everything we do like this, everything that destroys the living earth and takes us further and further from any natural feeling, is an externalization of our own imbalance. It does not improve the situation.

The key is to now bring the Energy back into our bodies. That's what this book is all about. Not to go back, not to give up what we have learned, not to repress or destroy the knowledge we have gained and the consciousness of which we have become capable. But to *grow* in physical energy, to grow in feeling, to strengthen the force of life in ourselves; to eat, finally, from the Tree of Life. This regaining of balance is the real meaning of health.

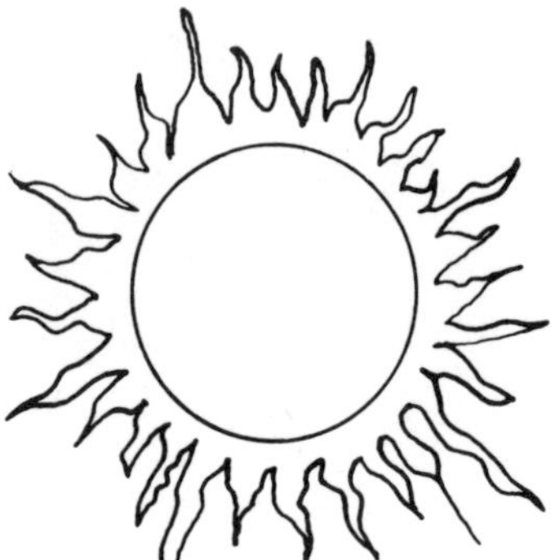

The vast majority of people today are not really happy, definitely not healthy, and living at only a small fraction of their potential. This is true for young and old, rich and poor, male and female. The miseries of mankind are terrifying in number and variety: physical, emotional, sexual, mental, social, political, economic, spiritual. There is no one who does not suffer from at least several of these kinds of problems—myself included. Nonetheless, there are some effective ways to deal with our difficulties and our personal tragedies. Restoring the full natural health and energy of the body, relaxing the grip of the conscious mind over the senses and emotions, and increasing your awareness of life and its power—these are three keys to dealing with everything.

An example. You're walking down a dark street late at night. You notice that several large men are following you, and you sense that the situation is dangerous. You become afraid. Immediately your heart starts to beat faster and your breathing gets shallower. Your legs feel weak; possibly your hands do too. You cannot think clearly, you cannot move easily. You haven't got much time before the men overtake you, but you are paralyzed by fear. What should you do?

Should you try to analyze the predicament and *think* of a way out? Try to escape by running blindly in some direction? Attempt to ignore your fears and keep on walking, hoping that nothing bad will happen? Maybe you should turn and attack your pursuers, regardless of the odds? Or should you just freeze and await the unknown in an unmoving panic?

None of these is very good as a first response. The first thing to do is to *relax.* Really. Relax body-and-mind, breathe as deeply and fully as possible, and try to center all your energy in the region of your hips and lower abdomen. (As will be explained later on, this region is the Hara, the body's center of gravity as well as the most unifying place for bodymind energy.) Only then will you be able to think clearly, and move swiftly and powerfully. Only then will you be able to deal with the situation in the most appropriate way.

The point is, first you've got to restore your inner balance by getting rid of fear and the immobilizing physical and mental results of fear. You've got to unite body-and-mind by concentrating everything at your physical center of movement and energy (the Hara)—and then act. Otherwise you may be defeating yourself before even meeting the situation!

I have seen hundreds of people utilizing this principle

in their daily lives. People who were having serious problems of various kinds—physical, emotional, sexual, even economic. By first paying attention to their health (their *psychosomatic* health, their body-mind health), they became able to handle difficulties that were previously destroying them. They gained the ability to maintain their balance and well-being even in adversity. And isn't that really the true test of health—and of character? In good times, in situations that are familiar and comfortable or at least not threatening, it's relatively easy to be relaxed, giving, warm, balanced, and centered. But to maintain that state of well-being in bad times, through dangers and troubles and setbacks, through illnesses and accidents and even in the face of death—that is real health. Most of us are a long way from it.

But then, what are we doing here? We are inhabitants of the planet Earth, tribesmen of the race of Man, members of some smaller families as father or mother, wife or husband, brother or sister, daughter or son. All of these identities carry responsibilities, burdens that may often seem heavy to bear. We must continue life. We must protect our loved ones. We must help those who suffer. We must renew the living world constantly, in the face of its constant destruction. None of this is easy.

There is another task, another duty, that really comes first in many respects: *coming to terms with yourself,* determining your own life needs and fulfilling them. It seems selfish, maybe. But it's a necessary selfishness, because only with good health and mental-emotional well-being can you proceed to live with other people in the best way, to give freely and without fear, to accomplish your work whatever it is, to use your energies in the most positive way.

The selfishness of attending to yourself is an investment that ultimately enables you to enrich the world and care for other people (besides just enjoying being alive) in a way that those who go on blindly, in poor or partial health, cannot do. It may be selfishness, but it's not laziness. *Health is hard work!* Five minutes of exercise a day won't do it. Seeing a psychiatrist once or twice a week won't do it. "Working out" strenuously every day, but spending the rest of your day the same way you did before—graceless, inactive, tense, fearful, negative, inflexible—won't do it either.

Health is a twenty-four-hour-a-day matter. It's relaxation, breathing, stretching, and moving like a beautiful animal. It's feeling deeply and not being afraid to show those feelings. It's fighting when necessary—but without hate. It's knowing Nature, as a child knows its mother—not as a conqueror. It's giving out your energy to others, yet remaining full. It's living *in this world,* beautifully.

What I am proposing in this book is quite simple in principle. Its achievement is mainly an individual affair. I have no "system" to propound, no set of rules, nothing to be bound by. I know this makes things harder, but I'd be dishonest if I tried to tell you what to eat, how to move, what to think, or how to live your life. I'm sorry there are so many "authorities" who *are* doing these things—and so many people following them! But I'm interested in you returning to your own senses, reclaiming your own body, opening up your own mind—not following me.

We humans seem to have two aspects: our old, primitive, animal nature, which is physical and instinctual, or "natural"; and our newer, historical, civilized nature, which is learned, intellectual, rational, technological—or "cultural." These two sides don't always get along very well. Most people's lives are marked by the subjugation of the natural by the cultural. The warring opposition of our two halves produces disease, confusion, shame, anxiety, tension, cruelty, exploitation, and other forms of unnatural pain.

The aim of this book is to help you bring these two halves of your own character together in some kind of new life. This would be a state of health that is not a compromise of nature or culture, but something greater that unites the two. It might be drawn like this:

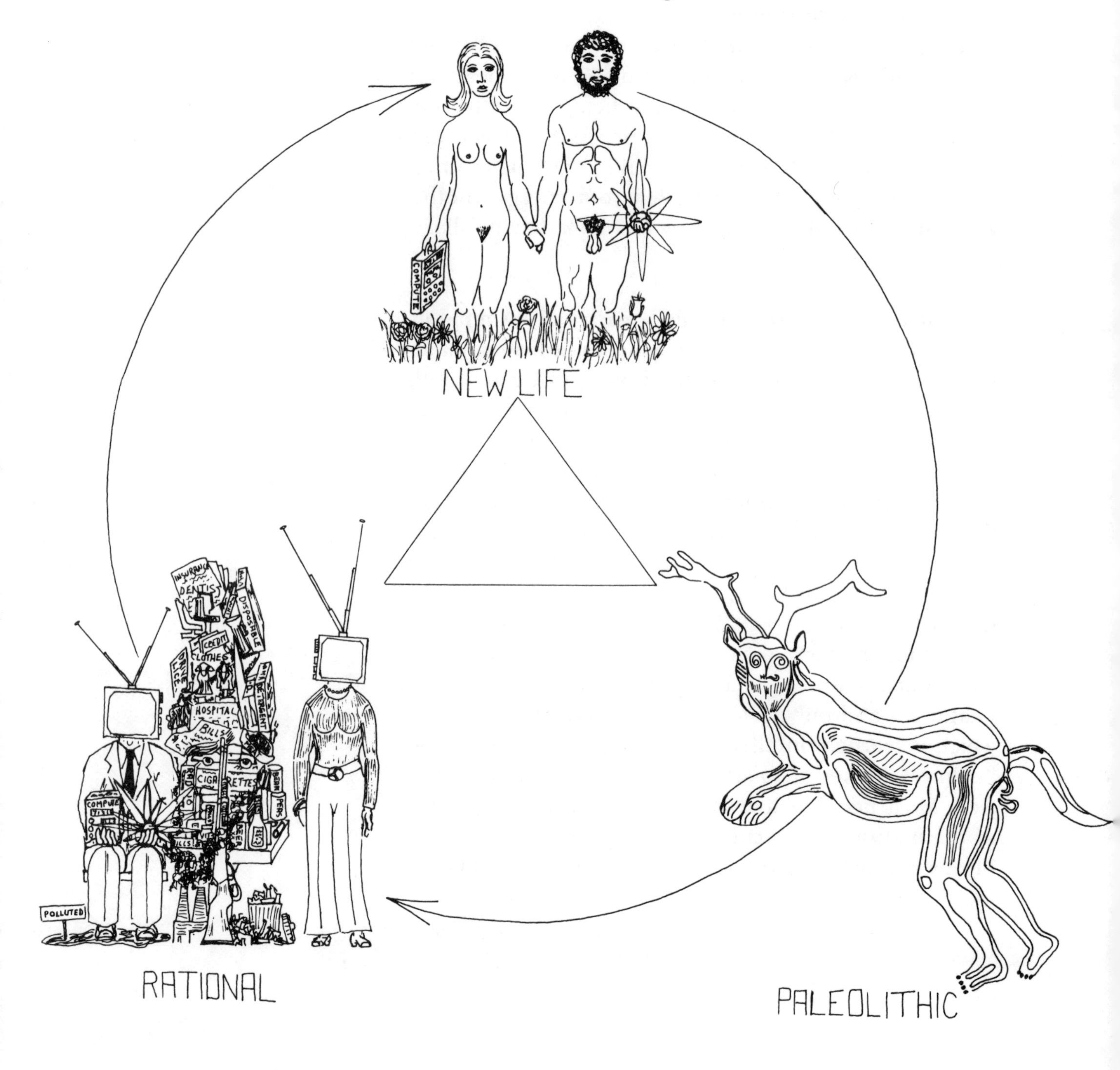

In this diagram I call the primal, animal life-energy in man the *Paleolithic* energy. Paleolithic is the Old Stone Age, dating from man's earliest appearance, up to about 10,000 years ago. I believe that the hunting-and-gathering peoples of this time, as well as those who have survived into modern times and still practice the old ways (such as the BaMbuti Pygmies of the Congo, the Eskimos and other hunting North American Indian tribes, and the Bushmen) were the last humans to manifest this energy in a pure form, in whole societies. Their way of life was physically demanding, for there was little in the way of technology to separate man from the harshness (and the beauty) of nature.

I call the modern, civilized aspect of man the *Rational,* because it is this form of thinking that most clearly differentiates man from the animals and creates the works of modern times: the social, political, economic structures and systems, the machinery, science, technology, culture, educational establishment, and mass media that dominate human life today. These are all products of the rational mind.

The Rational Era is the period of historical time, and it is coming to a close. It has to. Ecological destruction, overpopulation, wars, poverty, crime, and general human misery all demonstrate that the life of man must change. It just doesn't work for us to be so out of our senses, so divided from ourselves, from our fellow human beings and from nature. The war between our old and new parts has to end.

Here's a very graphic example. William Stekel once defined sexual impotence as a war between the spine and the brain. The spine is the "lower" instincts, ruled by the old brain (cerebellum) in all animals—including man; all nervous energy goes to and comes from all parts of the body via the spinal cord. The brain is the "higher" nature of man, ruled by the frontal lobes (cerebral cortex), which only man possesses in such large proportion; it is rational and abstract thought, ideas, images, language, societally-conditioned feelings and other mental patterns instilled by the educational system, literature, the mass media, and human culture. Okay, got that? The spine is instinct, the brain is thought. The spine is the body, the brain is the mind. The spine is nature within us, the brain is culture and history within us.

Now, Stekel says impotence is the result of a war, brain against spine. It has been proven that sexual impotence in the male is *almost never* a malfunction of purely physical origin. Less than one out of every hundred cases are caused by body problems such as the testicles failing to produce hormones in sufficient quantity, or some organic damage to the penis. In nearly every case it is some event in the *mind* that blocks the natural functioning of the male sex organs. Psychosomatic war—brain versus spine.

There is an "erection center" in the spine that controls the erectile mechanism of the penis. It is located just a few inches above the coccyx, or base of the spine. This center can be stimulated by touch (at the genitals or other sensitive areas), by erotic thoughts, by the sight of an attractive woman, by certain sounds or certain words, also by smell. But whatever causes the stimulation, the *nervous system* communicates this information to the erection center, which then produces an erection.

The central nervous system consists of the brain and the spine. The brain (specifically, the forebrain or cerebrum) is the seat of all our thoughts, fears, insecurities, guilt feelings, shame, anxiety, confusion, and other negative mental phenomena concerning sex. (Animals, on the other hand, lacking our splendid cerebral capacities, also lack any anxieties or inhibitions about sexual performance!) Under the influence of such negative thoughts and feelings, the brain can quite easily *veto* the action of the erection center. It can do this in two ways: either by cutting off the flow of stimulating information to the center (for example, by repressing your desire to have sex, because of social convention, personal inhibition, fear of rejection, or fear of failure); or by "jamming" the output *from* the already-stimulated center to the genital organs (the desire is there, but the erection ain't). In either case the result is impotence.

The problem is obviously not in the penis or testicles, but in the brain of their "owner." To solve the problem he *must* deal with the negative messages the brain is sending down the spine to destroy natural sexual functioning. Any method of treating impotence that does not treat the mind cannot possibly work. The brain must become the co-worker of the spine, not its enemy. (There are several successful ways in which this can be done—which will be discussed later.)

If we extend this same principle to include physical health in general, and in fact the whole life of man on this planet, the necessity of ending the war between brain and spine still holds true. Only now we can call them mind and life.

When we hear the word "health" we usually understand it to mean health of the body—freedom from illness, plenty of energy, grace and skill of movement, long life. But health of the body depends on health of the mind. By itself, your body works perfectly; it wants only to move, to breathe fresh air and drink clean water, to eat natural foods, to propagate itself, and to feel pleasure. But its natural movement, breathing, nourishment, and feeling are all distorted, restricted, polluted, and twisted by your mind. Your body is alive, it *is* life, it is the form that your spirit (don't you have a spirit, a soul, an essential spark of something?) takes to live on this earth. But your mind doesn't *necessarily* live; it can work for life, with life, or against it. We have to turn our minds to life. A force flows in our own bodies, and in all other living things—and we can reunite with it. *Mind fixed on life.* Think about it.

A few more things before we take off. Most people see the world as a two-way highway. You can either go one way or the other. If you're too fat, you go on a crash diet. If you're uptight or repressed, you get drunk or stoned, ride the other direction for a while, then sleep it off and go to work Monday morning the same as ever. Don't like the big, impersonal, corrupt and cruel government? Join a big, impersonal, corrupt movement for its overthrow. Bored and unhappy with your domestic sex life? Have an extramarital sex affair, which is bound to be just as boring and unhappy. This road you're on is too noisy, too fast, too full of fumes, too physically numbing to keep driving on, and you don't know where you're going anyhow? Well, they say, just turn around and drive the *other* way and everything'll be all right. But it ain't necessarily so!

What we do need is a lot more self-reliance. Get *off* the road and figure out what's wrong. Don't accept the idea that there are only two ways to go—there are a million!

Freedom is probably the hardest thing to live with. Some people don't even seem to want it at all. They like to have their lives defined for them by someone else. But some of us think things need changing, and we had better start with ourselves. This demands that we get rid of some preconceived ideas and established principles about the way things are or ought to be—that we lay aside the masks that others see us in, give up the disguises and the games and the array of false securities that keep us from facing ourselves, from seeing our own lives without deception. And be left with—what?

Nothing to rely on. No maps of the way. No one to follow but yourself. Don't be afraid! You already have everything you need! All the wisdom and the power and the love is waiting inside you, to be opened up, set free, and used to live. It's not easy. It's hard work. But what more important work have you got to do?

No one can really free a slave, except the slave himself. No one can *make* you healthy and fully alive—but you yourself. Oh yes, you can improve things somewhat by following one health system or another (or one after another, as many people do), but it's not real health if you don't get there yourself.

Freedom and health arc much the same thing. You can go to a good doctor or a good psychiatrist or a good guru or follow a good diet—and be like some zoo animal who's given the right amount of food every day, a little exercise, and perhaps kept alive quite a while without any serious illness. Except for the illness of living in a cage. Except for the diseases of not knowing yourself, not being in touch with your own deepest feelings and your own body, not being in control of your own existence. You might appear healthy, yet not be free to grow and change and live as you really want to live.

Or you can say *yes* to yourself and, with the help of this book or without it, stop the war inside you, determine for yourself what's necessary and what isn't, what's good and what isn't—and get down to some real living.

Declare your health and independence! "This is my body and my brain—no one else's. The responsibility for their functioning and their balance is mine—no one else's. And the struggle to live well, starting right now, and to grow further, is mine—and no one else's."

Accepting this responsibility for ourselves, this centeredness, we can begin to give and take in the world, and to live well with others. Self-reliant health is really the freedom to live at the center of the universe, because that center is everywhere. It's where you are, right now.

This is my gospel, the "good news" of real health, which is the reunification of body and mind in the *body-mind* of a new life: like the Kingdom of Heaven, it is all within you!

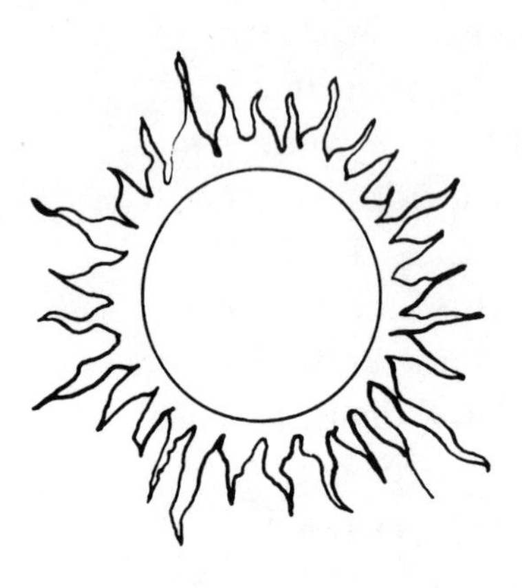

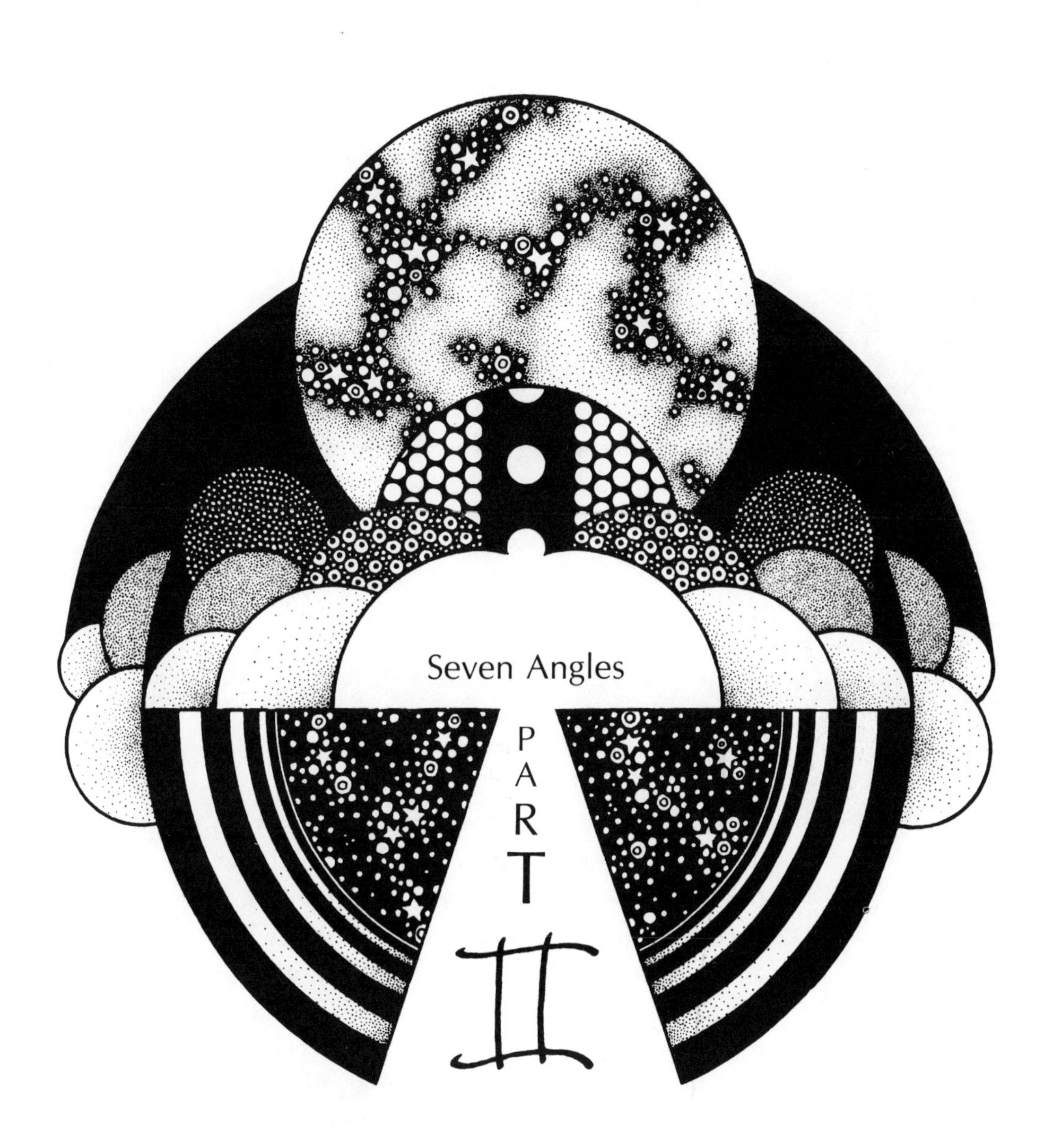
Seven Angles
PART
II

MOVE!

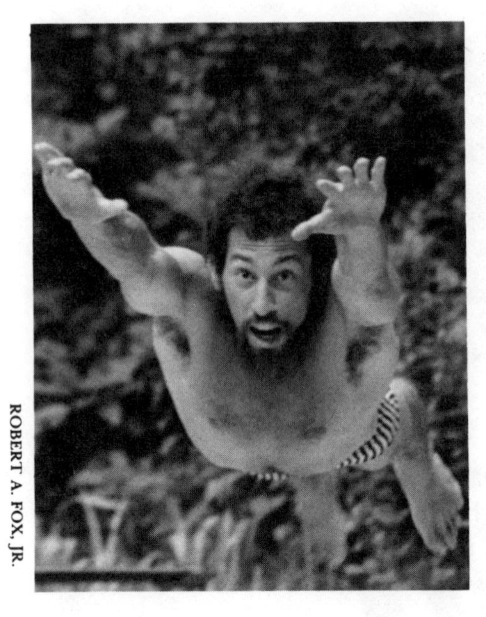

ROBERT A. FOX, JR.

Life is a dance, a game, a song, a road, a river, a maze, a battle! Get up and dance it, sing, jump, walk, crawl, climb, soar, fight, play, run, *move!* All that lives, moves! But you sit too much, you sigh and watch a healthy life slip by, bemoaning your unhappy state, when your body itself wants to move, needs to move, was made to move! Put the book down, let yourself go. You can do it—move!

> The living organism . . . is alive because it moves.
>
> ALEXANDER LOWEN, *Pleasure*

You are built to move all day long, eat enough to keep going, sleep soundly even on rough ground, get up with the sun and move again. Your whole array of bones, muscles, joints, and organs is no different from that of Stone Age man and woman, who hunted wild animals and gathered wild fruits and plants and fought off predators all day long—except that you use them less! When you were born you weren't any less well-endowed for movement than a child of the Masai tribesmen of East Africa, who can run 40 miles every day; you weren't any less well-equipped than a baby of the Tarahumara Indians of Mexico, who run 200-mile nonstop kickball races over rocky mountain terrain, for fun! The human body is a machine built for movement, for action, for energy. Life *is* movement!

Movement keeps your body alive:

1. It stimulates the circulation of blood and *strengthens* the heart.
2. It deepens and regulates breathing and clears the lungs.
3. It charges the nervous system.
4. It massages and strengthens the internal organs as well as the external muscles.
5. It activates the all-important endocrine glands.
6. It improves your mental capacities.
7. And, invariably, healthy movement stimulates your body and mind in such a way as to actually *give* you more energy than you expend!

Strenuous exercise also produces sweating, which clears your body of poisonous wastes. And if you can keep up the exertion level for some length of time (like a 20-minute run), then your heart and lungs are strengthened remarkably, your endurance is increased, and your ability to absorb life-giving oxygen from the air can be permanently improved. So keep moving!

This book is going to suggest a lot of different kinds of movement, exercise, and physical practices. And I hope you try them out—don't just sit and read about them. We live in a society where everyone sits and lets the machines do the work. The antidote to this sickness is plenty of movement. No amount of proper movement is too much! *But:* You have to start slowly, especially if you've been sitting for a long time and haven't felt the ease and pleasure of moving your body well since you were a child. Your mind is stronger than your body, and it can lead you astray. If, after years of indolence, cigarette smoking, and sedentary work, you suddenly decide that you should exercise, and you dash out and try to run five miles—you may get into some trouble. Don't try to direct things so much. Learn to listen to your body. When you *feel* like moving—that's when you should move.

How do you *know* when to move, how strenuously, and when to stop? There is no formula to follow. You learn only by doing, and that's why you have to start slowly. Start with a very brisk walk, or a slow jog—just 5 or 10 minutes' worth. Stop, relax, see how you feel. Next day, you can build on what you have learned. After a while you will get a very good idea of what your body needs for good condition, and what's too much for it.

The inertia and disease of years of inactive, unhealthy living is like the muddy sediment at the bottom of a pond. It can be flushed out—no matter what age you are—but not all at once. Vigorous movement is like clear water rushing into the long-stagnant pond; it stirs up the mud quite a bit at first. A heavy dose of exercise may start more of your sedimented past moving than you care to feel. Heavy smokers, for example, who decide to try running a couple of miles will discover that the sustained deep-breathing that a good run requires will stir up some pretty nasty stuff from their lower lungs. They may feel pains in the chest, ribs, diaphragm, back, and stomach. Argh! Actually, it's probably a good pain—but it should be taken in small doses.

What might a "good" pain be? Good pain is when you stretch out a tight muscle. Good pain is when your little heart pounds away at 130, 140, or more beats per minute during a hard run. Good pain is blood coursing into a muscle complex that has been long unused. It's the flexing of a stiff spinal column. It's blowing your nose, it's fasting, it's climbing a mountain. Good pain is any discomfort you feel that is caused by a *beneficial* flow of energy, a healing or cleansing process.

The discomfort of "good" pain is an index of how far that muscle or organ or joint has been allowed to lapse from its healthy condition. At first you may have to remind yourself that something may be good for you even though it hurts. You might be doing a yoga stretching exercise, for example, and say to yourself: "This discomfort in the back of my leg is merely the result of an overly taut hamstring muscle being stretched out in a slow and completely safe manner, so don't worry about it." After a while, though, your senses will return as you become reacquainted with your body and learn to understand its language a bit better. Then you'll be able to tell the difference immediately between a healthy, benefical discomfort and real or "bad" pain.

Real pain is a danger signal. When you cut yourself, or break a bone, or come down with a serious illness, something has to be done about it. You feel pain in order to be made aware of a threat to your health and safety, so that you can turn the forces of your conscious and unconscious energies to the task of healing. After some time you won't be likely to confuse these danger signals with the feelings of "good" pain—which actually won't "hurt" so much, but will instead be almost welcomed as signs of improvement.

I like to talk about movement rather than exercise. "Exercise" usually connotes a defined, predetermined, limited set of prescribed movements, done in an orderly fashion to improve your strength, speed, flexibility, endurance, coordination, or whatever. Push-ups, sit-ups, a one-mile run, a tennis game, a wrestling practice, a weightlifting workout—all are exercise. They're fine, but not enough. Real bodymind health is the result of a pattern of moving, and living, that applies 24 hours a day.

Here's a good example. Drop this book on the floor, then pick it up. Observe how you do it. Observe how other people pick things up off the floor. It's usually done by bending forward from the waist, keeping your legs straight, or almost straight, and using only your lower back muscles. Right?

There's a much more graceful, natural, and interesting way to do it. Try this: Keeping your back vertical (or almost), bend your knees deeply, lowering your *whole* body toward the floor until you are in a crouched or squatting position, with one foot slightly ahead of the other. The leading foot should be flat on the floor,

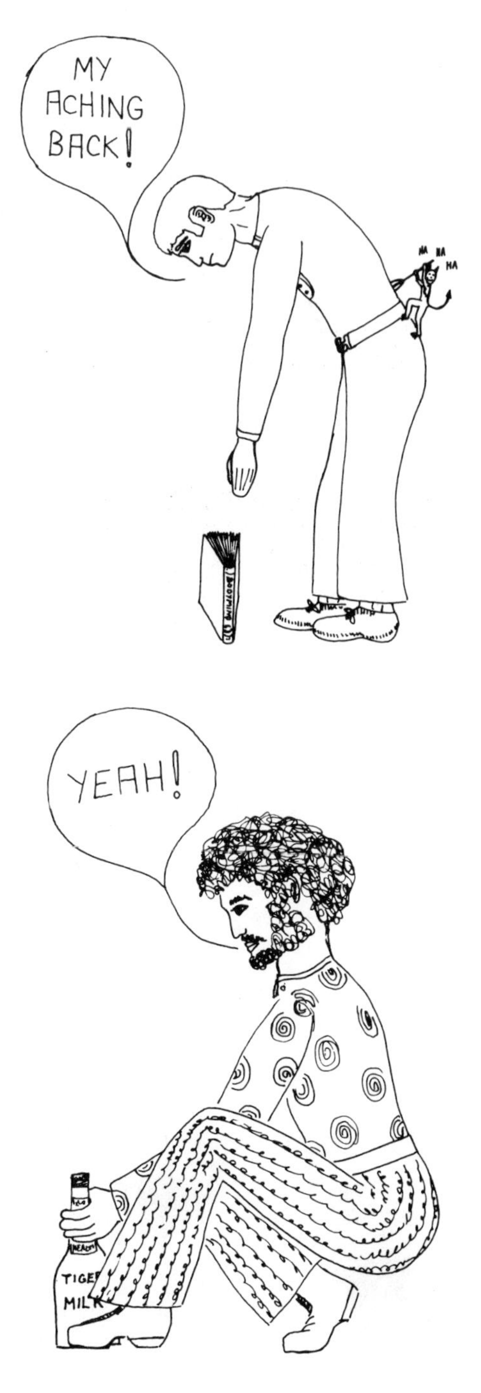

the rear foot should have the heel off the ground. Then rise by using the large muscles of your thighs, buttocks, and calves, keeping the spine erect. Do it a few times, then do it the other way and *feel* the difference.

You may be a little uncomfortable crouching instead of bending over—that's "good" pain! It results from a lack of flexibility in your hip joints, knees, or ankles; from physical top-heaviness; or from general lack of strength in the lower half of your body. But moving this way improves your flexibility and increases your leg strength—and in a while it will become quite easy (even pleasurable!). Look at someone else trying the two ways, or at yourself in the mirror. The kneeling-crouching movement is powerful, smooth, and beautiful—and always well-balanced and "centered." Also this is the *only* way to lift very heavy things from the ground without strain and potential damage to the lower back, as anyone who works regularly with heavy objects can tell you.

Probably most of your everyday movements could be similarly altered for the better—but rather than suggesting the changes to you, I'd like you to discover them for yourself. Your body is constantly sending you messages—become aware of them and pay attention! It's not enough, you see, to embark on some diet or exercise program, no matter how strenuous, if the rest of the day you ignore your body, sit slumped over, breathe shallowly, don't take breaks from your work for just plain freedom of movement, and generally keep your natural energies bottled up. *It's got to be a constant, continual way of being, not something you "do" at certain times.*

This book is going to be a waste of your time if you just sit and read it. A lot of statements are made here which are not meant to *convince* you of anything. The only way you can know what I'm talking about is to try it. This chapter is about movement, and before we go on any further, I am asking you to get up and move.

Specifically, I'd like you to stretch and bend and flex your body for a few minutes (with as few clothes on as possible); then do at least 10 full minutes of some natural activity like running, swimming, jogging, hiking, uninhibited dancing, or fast walking—without stopping to rest. It is very important, for reasons I'll explain when you get back, that the action be continuous. So if you get tired and can't keep going, don't stop altogether but slow down a bit, and pick it up again when you can.

I'm very serious about this. If you're an 80-year-old woman and it's the dead of winter, you can still bundle up and take a nice half-mile walk. (Our ancestors did a lot more, and their lives depended on it. So do ours.) Ten minutes is not much to ask—and I know you'll feel better for it!

If you can possibly get outdoors for this, do so. But make sure you either go to a park, or along an untraveled road, or best of all, somewhere in the country. You don't want to be out jogging down 42nd Street during rush hour, sucking in huge lungfuls of carbon monoxide and automobile fumes and dust and dirt and polluted air when you need oxygen. If you can't get outdoors to some reasonable place with some reasonably good air, try a gym or a swimming pool—or just run and dance around your own room. But make sure you do at least 10 minutes without stopping. Okay?

Do it alone. Some nice sociable sport such as tennis or handball might seem like a good substitute, but the solitary experience is vital. So, my friend, please put down the book now (fascinating as it may be), stretch out, get into some comfortable old clothes, and *do it.*

There are different kinds of movement, and they all affect you in different ways. What you have just done (I hope) is a form of *aerobic* exercise.

Literally, aerobic means "with oxygen." Whenever you move, your body must use up more oxygen than it requires in a resting state, in supplying the energy for that movement. More oxygen can be delivered to your body in two ways: by taking more air into your lungs each minute, and by increasing your heart rate (beats per minute). If your exertion (jogging, for example) doesn't raise your body's demands for oxygen higher than can be met in these two ways, and therefore you can *maintain* the exertion over an extended period of time, it is called "aerobic." By working your heart and lungs a little more than usual, you can maintain a "steady-state" for quite a while, in which you are taking in as much oxygen as you need to keep going. This "state," though, involves much higher energy-expenditure than your normal activities—and inactivities.

Stated more simply: Aerobic exercise is anything you do that requires more oxygen than you normally use, but *not* more than you can get by stepping up your heartbeat and air intake. Thus you can keep up the activity for some time without tiring.

Your lungs take the oxygen from the air you breathe and deliver it to the heart, which sends it through the bloodstream to your muscles, where it is used to burn foodstuffs to produce energy. The lungs can *increase* the amount of oxygen they send to the heart in three ways:

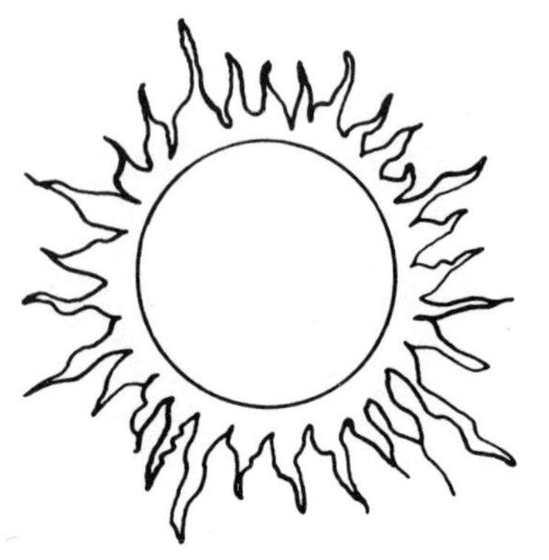

1. By taking in more air on each breath. "Vital capacity" is the total volume of air you can breathe out after the deepest inhale you can take. The average adult's vital capacity is five quarts—yet the average breath taken during normal activity is only half a quart! During strenuous exertion of the aerobic type, a single breath may contain 60 percent of the vital capacity, or three quarts. This is six times the normal breath. Quite an improvement!
2. By increasing the breathing rate. During exercise the breathing may become four or five times faster than normal. (Normal for an adult is 10 to 12 breaths per minute.)

These first two factors alone can increase the amount of

fresh air taken into the lungs each minute by a factor of 20 or more! Obviously, this means the amount of oxygen available is *20 times* as much. The average resting "pulmonary ventilation" (amount of air inhaled and exhaled) is about five to six quarts per minute. A short spell of hard exercise can take this up as high as 150 quarts per minute, or more; but for the prolonged, aerobic steady-state exercise, the maximal pulmonary ventilation is 80 to 100 quarts per minute.

3. By increasing the lungs' ability to absorb oxygen from any given amount of air. In other words, the lungs' efficiency improves. This is one part of the "training effect," which only becomes evident after aerobic exercise has been continued regularly over a long period of time.

The primary benefits of aerobic activity are to the cardiovascular and respiratory systems. Your heart gets stronger, your circulation improves, your arteries are kept from hardening, your lungs become more efficient, your breathing pattern deepens. Secondary benefits include improved digestion (more oxygen becomes available for the digestive process, which means you can obtain more nutrients from the same amount of food); better muscle tone and skin tone; and generally having a lot more energy. But these effects don't take place overnight—and they don't come without plenty of hard work and "good" pain!

Anyone who claims you can get healthy on a 60-second exercise plan, or with some fancy machine that "does the work for you," or just on some special diet with no movement required, is selling you a dangerously false bill of goods. Without some form of aerobic exercise at least three or four times a week, your heart and lungs cannot be in really healthy condition—and they're the two most important organs in your body.

Also, aerobic activity strengthens the will and clears the mind. When you're running five miles on a winding country road early in the morning, breathing deeply and steadily, feeling the rhythm and form of your stride, the coordination of breath and step, drinking in the beauty

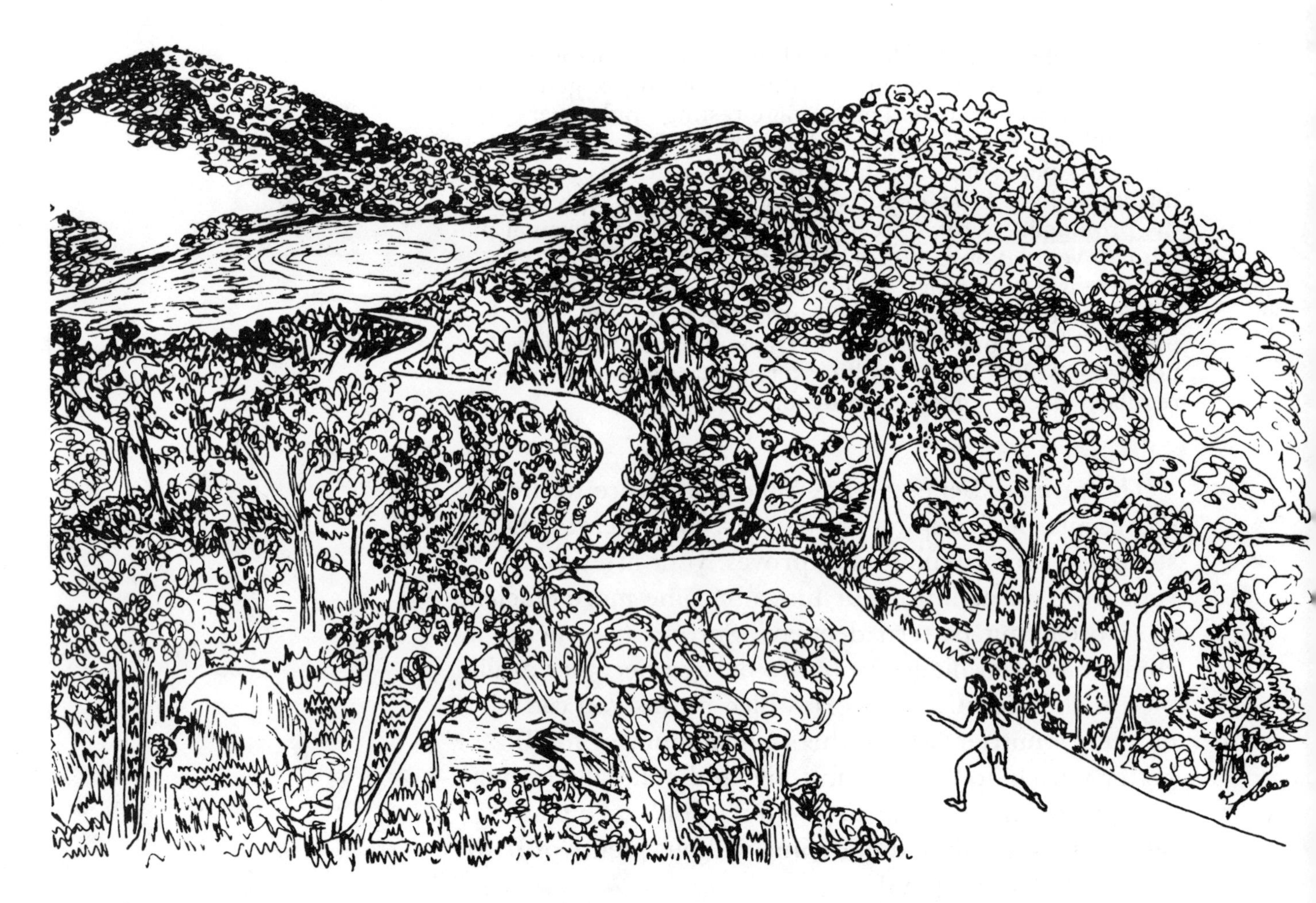

of the woods in the morning—then you can't really *think* about too much else. You can't worry, you can't plan, you just concentrate on the running. You get into a state of meditation-in-motion.

I don't want to tell you too much about the effects all this has on your mind. They're amazing, but you'll have to experience them yourself. Put on them running shoes, brothers and sisters, and you'll see what I mean!

Any vigorous activity that demands more oxygen than you customarily consume, but not more than you can take in (and maintain this intake in a prolonged steady-state), is aerobic. The most common, natural movements, employing large sections of your total body musculature, are by far the best—running, swimming, hiking, cycling, jogging, dancing, making love.

These are all *rhythmic* actions, characterized by alternate contractions and relaxations of the muscles involved. In running, for example, the hamstring muscle contracts to pull your leg back, powering the stride, then relaxes as you swing the leg forward. This rhythmicity is a valuable quality in movement of any kind. When a muscle contracts to do work, it sets up a demand for oxygen and other nutrients in the muscle tissue. But the flow of blood carrying these nutrients to the muscle is restricted, and may even be cut off completely, by the strong contraction. Not until the muscle relaxes again can fresh blood flow freely into the muscle, deliver its supplies, and carry off waste products such as carbon dioxide and water. Then the rhythm continues, with another contraction.

In another sense rhythmicity is important on emotional and psychic levels. All life follows rhythmic patterns: the cycles of the seasons, the alternations of day and night, our own internal rhythms of heartbeat, breathing cycle, brain waves. By moving your body rhythmically, you "tune in" with the patterns of the natural world and feel more a part of the natural order of things. A good way to feel!

So aerobic activity improves your health in a lot of ways. I consider my daily run or swim to be *the* most important part of the day. It's the one thing I do that really brings body, mind, and spirit together—and strengthens all of them. And, provided you start slowly and always listen to your body's communications, it is virtually impossible to overdo aerobic activity. (Remember the Tarahumara and their three-day nonstop kickball races.) Start now, and your health will improve tremendously, with no end in sight! Perhaps, early on some misty morning, we will meet down one of those back country roads.

All activity that isn't aerobic is *anaerobic*—which literally means "without oxygen." Either these are activities that 1) don't require much more oxygen than the resting state (like slow walking); or 2) *do* require more oxygen, but your lungs and heart can't provide it so no steady-state is ever reached, and you cut the action short—either voluntarily (you stop) or involuntarily (you drop). Short spurts of violent activity, such as sprint running, fast swimming, and weight lifting, fall into this second category.

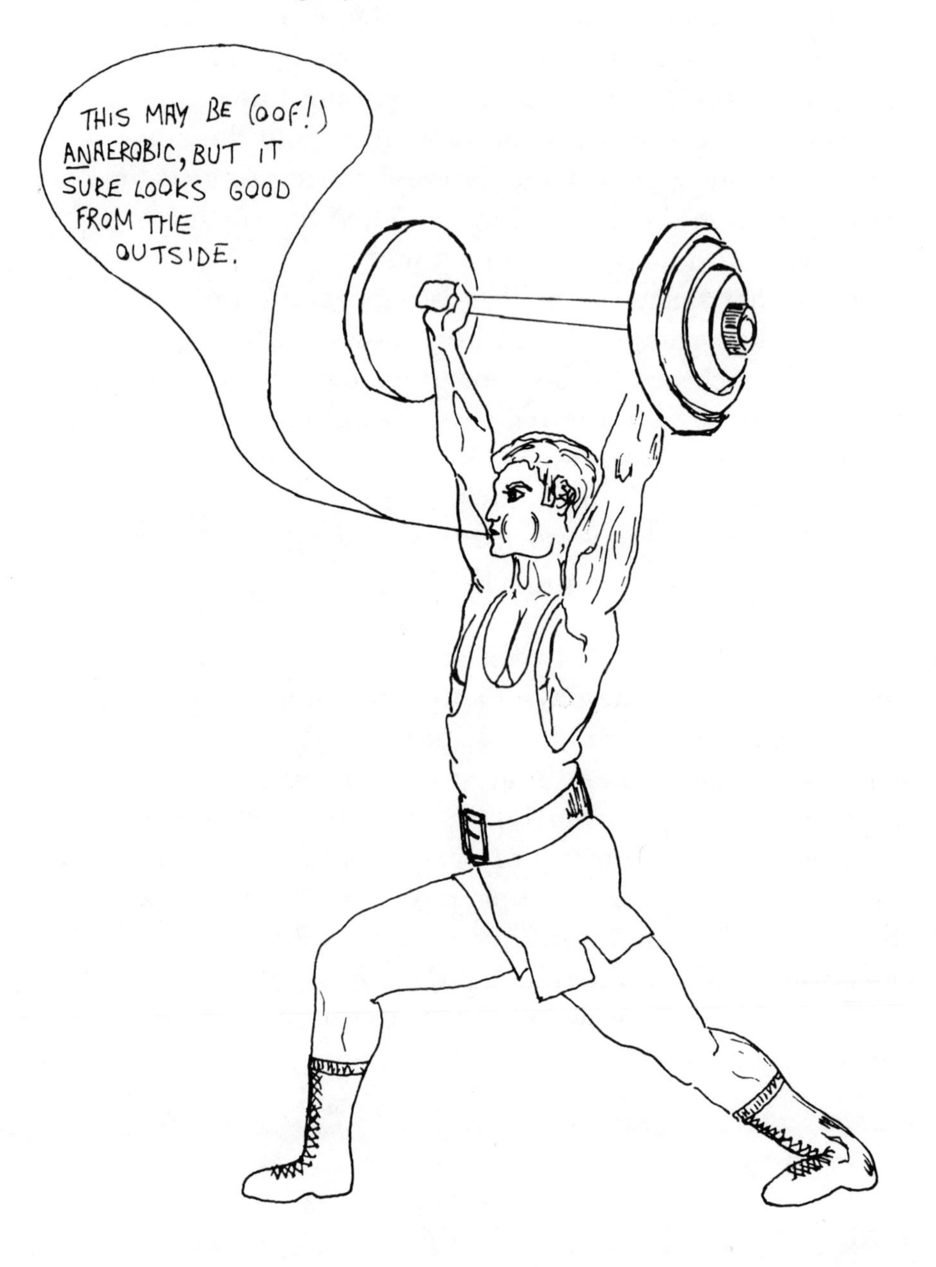

Activities of this second type build up an "oxygen debt": That is, the body temporarily supplies the required energy in ways that don't use so much oxygen. But this creates a great strain within your system, and the oxygen imbalance soon has to be corrected—by stopping or slowing down, panting, breathing heavily, and reducing your effort until a recovery is effected.

Anaerobic movements come in many forms, with different results. They can promote flexibility, strength, coordination, balance, speed, power, grace of movement, sensitivity, better circulation, self-awareness, and lots more. Anaerobic activity is essential to healthy living, just as aerobic activity is.

For example, full-speed sprint running has many advantages over long-distance aerobic running. It strengthens the hip, leg, and torso muscles (particularly the calf, hamstring, and buttock muscles) in a way that the shorter, slower stride of easy distance running cannot do. Sprinting also raises your heart rate into the over-150 beats per minute range, which is very good for your cardiovascular and circulatory condition—*provided* that your heart has been trained to take the strain, gradually and over a long period of time.

Sprinting also demands, and produces, greater flexibility of the lower back, ankles, and hip joints—which otherwise stay stiff and deadened in most people. Finally, running at top speed gives you a feeling of grace and power, the natural "high" of exerting your energies to the fullest—which most of us in "civilized" societies rarely experience. It's a good feeling.

There are dozens of anaerobic activities, including most sports, martial arts, dance techniques, yoga systems, sensory-awareness methods, as well as the traditional calisthenics and weight training. Since you've already been convinced of the necessity for some kind of aerobic exercise on a daily basis, why not add some anaerobic training as well? Try sprinting that last 100 yards. Feel the blood pound in your veins, feel your natural energies being released as they haven't been for a long time. Everyone should do this. And since you've been sitting still reading this for long enough, now's a good time for you to get up—and MOVE!

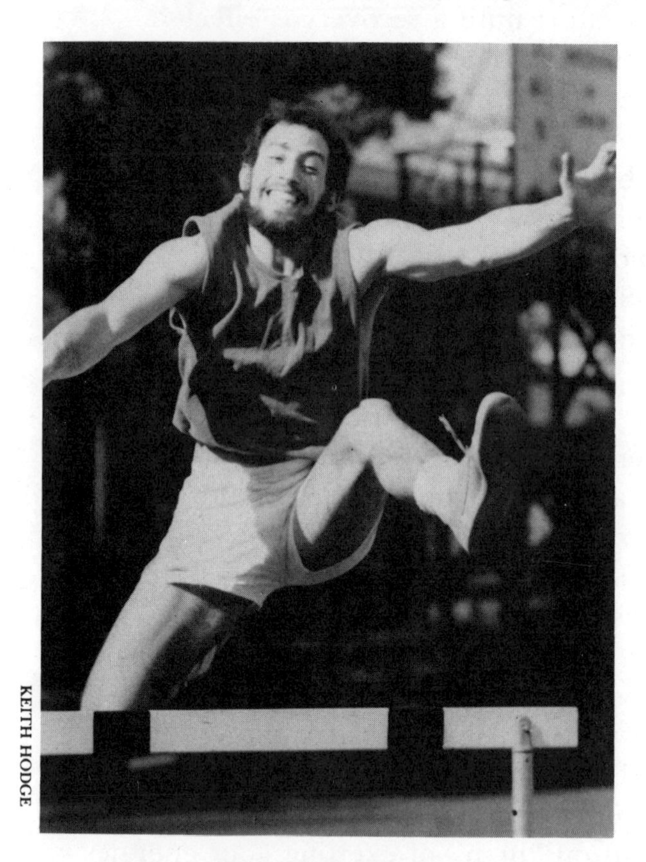

KEITH HODGE

The author's brother overcoming an obstacle

BREATH IS LIFE

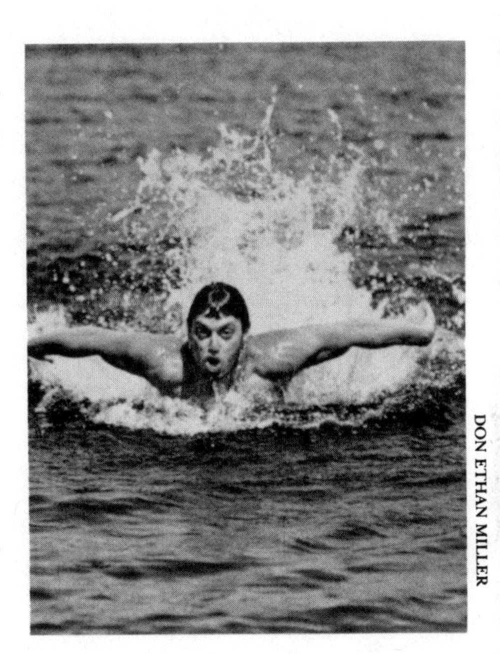

DON ETHAN MILLER

Life starts with a breath
and ends with the end of breath.

YOGI BHAJAN

You'll probably agree that breathing is the most important physical function of every living animal. But are you aware of your own breathing pattern? Probably more physical and mental disorders today are caused by poor breathing than by any other factor; see how you do.

Observe your own breathing. Put down the book, keeping your posture and body position the same; close your eyes. Don't change your breathing pattern, just observe it, bring it to your consciousness. Check the following characteristics:

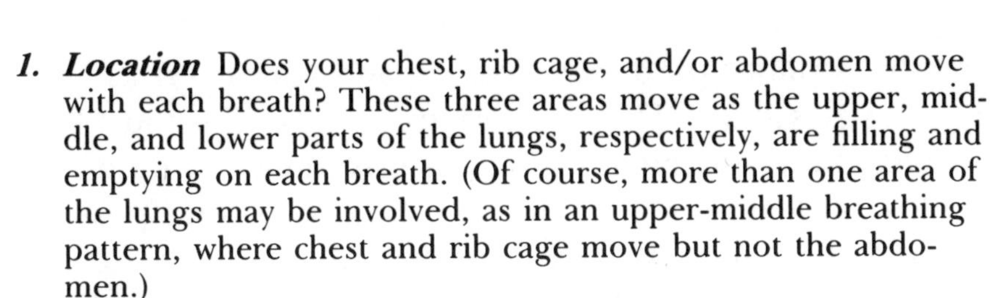

1. ***Location*** Does your chest, rib cage, and/or abdomen move with each breath? These three areas move as the upper, middle, and lower parts of the lungs, respectively, are filling and emptying on each breath. (Of course, more than one area of the lungs may be involved, as in an upper-middle breathing pattern, where chest and rib cage move but not the abdomen.)
2. ***Volume*** Would you say your breathing is shallow, medium, or deep? Of the total volume of air your lungs can hold, what percentage would you say is moving in and out with each breath?
3. ***Rhythm*** About how many times per minute do you breathe? Is this a regular rhythm or does it change often, with a series of shorter breaths being followed by several longer ones?
4. ***Nose or mouth*** Are you breathing through your nose or

your mouth? Or in through your nose and out through your mouth, or vice versa?

5. ***Nasal passages*** If all or part of your breathing is through your nose, does the air flow evenly and clearly through both nostrils at the same time, or only through one, or more through one than the other? Are the nasal passages completely clear or are they obstructed with mucus, dust, or some other stuff? If your breathing is all or partly through the mouth, is this because your nasal passages are obstructed?

You may find yourself becoming self-conscious when trying to check these factors, so that you change your breathing pattern as soon as you turn your attention to it. (Such delightful tricks the mind can play!) You can avoid this, though, by catching yourself at different times of the day and checking your breathing then: on a bus, at work, upon rising, after eating, and so on. After a while you'll have a good picture of your breathing pattern and its changes. While you're at it, check out some other people's breathing habits as well, with respect to the same five qualities—you may be surprised at what you find! (Most people, it is alarming to report, barely breathe at all. Perhaps they're robots?)

Most of us have been taught that breathing is an event that takes place in the chest. "Take a deep breath" is understood to mean "expand your chest as much as possible." This is a serious mistake. For most people, chest breathing, or "upper breathing," is the shallowest, least efficient, and least healthy pattern possible. This is especially true for women, whose chest cavities are rarely as large, relative to body size, as those of men. Yet the vast majority of women in civilized society breathe almost exclusively in the chest. But if you observe very young children, or primitive people living healthy outdoor lives, or even most civilized types when they are deep asleep, you will never see this shallow chest breathing!

Middle or rib-cage breathing is usually found in combination with either partial-upper or partial-lower breathing patterns. In either case it is deeper and healthier than chest breathing alone. Many active men in our culture—laborers, craftsmen, farmers, athletes—breathe mainly in this way.

Lower or abdominal breathing is superior to either chest or rib-cage breathing alone—yet it is hardly ever seen among adults in our society, except those with special training. This is the way children, "primitives," and deep sleepers breathe. Although you do not actually breathe with your abdomen, your belly moves outward with every inhale, inward with every exhale, and the associated downward-upward movement of the diaphragm fills and empties your lower lungs. In the other two forms of breathing, no fresh air reaches the lower lungs at all.

Abdominal breathing is the most natural form. It moves more air through the lungs than the other two patterns. And it also cleans the lungs of the sediment of smoke, air pollutants, and other impurities that otherwise may remain there for years. Middle and upper breathers have a large "residual volume" of air (in the lower lungs) that doesn't move—this is where most of those nasty old impurities reside. But with lower breathing no such residual volume exists, because the air passes through the upper and middle lungs en route to and from the lower lungs. Makes sense, doesn't it?

Here's how to do abdominal breathing: Lie on your back, on a firm surface such as a rug or hard mattress (the floor is fine; the earth itself is best). Be sure your clothing is *very* loose around your waist. Try to get your spine flat on the ground (instead of arched), bringing your knees up and placing the soles of your feet on the floor will help. Raise your head slightly, with a pillow or your hands, so that you can see your chest and stomach. Now exhale as completely as you can, through your mouth, making sure your chest collapses, rib cage contracts, and belly falls inwards as your upper, middle, and lower lungs (respectively) empty of air.

Begin to inhale, slowly (through either nose or mouth is okay for now), *making your belly rise.* Chest, rib-cage, and shoulders should not move at all—only the abdomen swells, as the lower lungs fill with air. You may find this very hard to accomplish at first, because it's exactly the opposite of the kind of breathing you were taught in schools, in gym classes, and at home. In abdominal breathing your stomach goes *out* on the inhale, is sucked *in* on the exhale.

If you are having trouble breathing this way, the best thing to do is just concentrate on relaxing your body and mind completely. Abdominal breathing is difficult to maintain when you are tense or anxious or *trying* very hard to achieve something (even abdominal breathing!). It occurs by itself often, during periods of rest, relaxation, pleasure, and familiarity—in fact, imagining that you are falling asleep will make it much easier for you to breathe this way. Another method is to place a light book or your hands on your belly, and push it up slightly, with each inhale.

Keep inhaling until your belly feels full and stretched; then exhale slowly, allowing it to fall inwards. Empty your lungs of as much air as you can—contract your abdominal muscles slightly at the end of the exhale to pull your stomach in and force every last bit of air out. After a short pause begin the whole cycle again. Repeat it at least 10 times.

When you can do this well, after several practices, try to maintain abdominal breathing while sitting, standing, and walking. Try to make a habit of it—it's superior to the upper breathing patterns in many ways. And it is the indispensable basis for the most healthy breathing pattern of all—Complete Breathing.

Complete Breathing is a basic Yogic practice and figures in several other health systems. Essentially, it is the filling and emptying of the lower, middle, and upper lungs in one long, wave-like motion. It combines chest, rib-cage, and abdominal breathing and is therefore the deepest form of breathing possible. It brings the most oxygen to the body with the least effort, benefits all the internal organs, and gives you a great feeling of well-being. The full value of Complete Breathing will not be evident until it has become second nature to you and is done without conscious effort. It can be practiced lying, sitting, or standing—but only *after* you have mastered abdominal breathing.

Complete Breathing

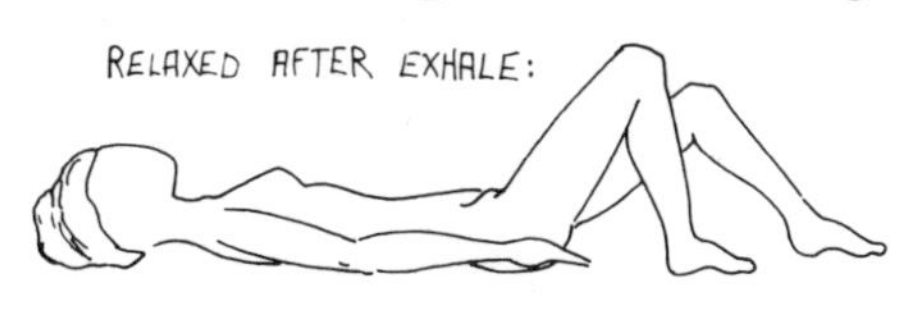

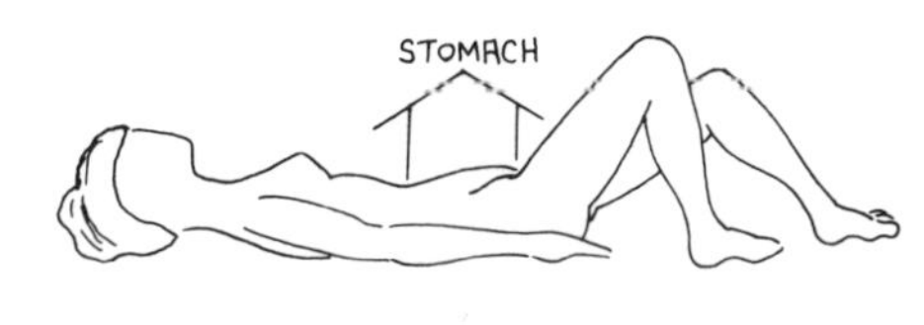

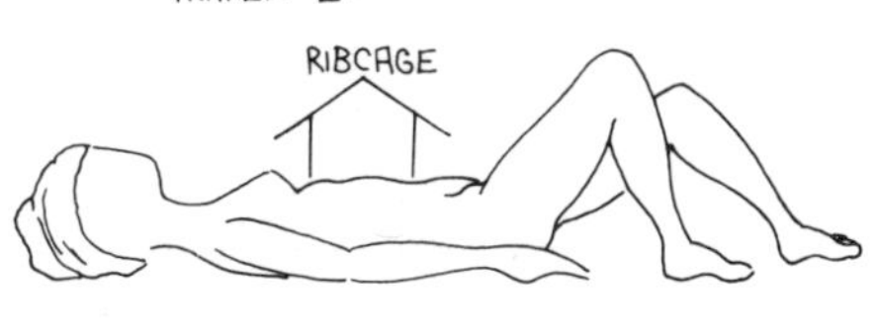

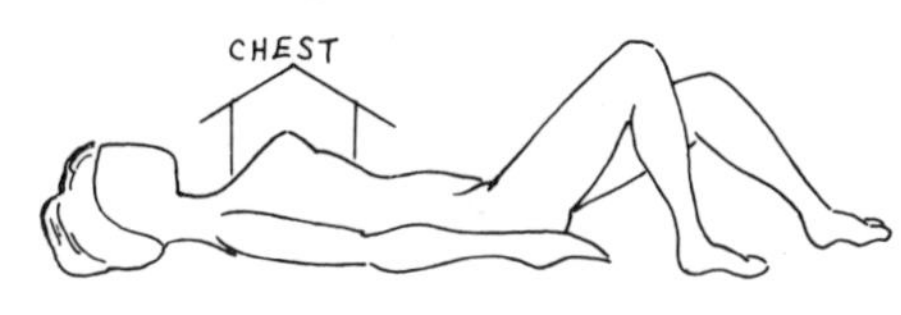

Relax and exhale as completely as possible. Start filling your lower lungs as you did in the abdominal breath. But when you feel about two-thirds full in the abdomen, allow the breath to rise to the ribs, which should expand outward, filling the middle lungs; and finally to the chest, which should expand fully, filling the upper lungs. This is the wave-like motion: *belly to rib-cage to chest.* (When the chest is filling, your stomach will again draw inwards, because your diaphragm has to move upwards to fill the upper lungs.)

Continue inhaling until you have drawn in as much air as you can comfortably hold; pause for a few seconds with your lungs full; then exhale, slowly. The exhalation is done in reverse order: *chest to rib-cage to belly.* Again, force the last bit of air out by contracting your abdominal muscles slightly. Pause for only a second, then begin the cycle again. This is Complete Breathing.

I mentioned in the last chapter that the volume of air moved by the average adult on each breath is about half a quart. This figure corresponds to the shallow chest-breathing pattern. With abdominal breathing, or even with deep chest-breathing, this can be doubled. With

Complete Breathing you can regularly take in three or even four quarts of air with each breath—six or eight times what you're probably getting now! More air means more oxygen, which, as in aerobic training, means better heart and lung condition, more complete digestion, improved mental functioning, and a lot more.

Another factor in healthy breathing is the balance between inhale and exhale. Some people tend to keep their lungs relatively full of air all the time, never exhaling completely. They perpetually keep a "reserve" quantity of air in their lungs (it may be as much as one-half the vital capacity of the lungs!), which is, of course, physiologically useless. Then there are other people who hardly ever inhale deeply and fully. They keep their lungs depressed, half-collapsed all the time. What is fascinating about these two kinds of incomplete breathers is that they frequently seem to be related to two kinds of neurotic emotional character traits.

People who cannot inhale deeply tend to be those who are *afraid to demand their right to live* fully, freely, and independently. They suffer from a neurotic fear of self-assertion and positive action; they lack confidence and healthy aggressiveness. They are afraid to take what they need to live.

People who cannot exhale completely tend to be those who are *afraid of letting go,* afraid of giving up their desperate hold on a rigid self-image, afraid of expressing their true feelings. Shouting, sobbing, sighing, laughing, screaming—these are all major exhalations that demand that you "let it out." People who cannot exhale are likely to be those who cannot let it out—they keep a tight, conscious hold on their feelings, thoughts, and actions—because they fear losing control over themselves.

Breathing practice for people such as these is not just an exercise to improve bodily health. It touches far deeper chords of a psychological, emotional, even spiritual nature. This is why all the great Asian systems of self-development—Yoga, Zen, Sufism, T'ai Chi, Karate, Aikido—lay such great stress on breathing. The Chinese say, "He who masters breathing can walk on the sand without leaving footprints." At the least, better breathing can give you a healthier, fuller, and longer life. Try it and see for yourself.

As we've seen, improved breathing gives you more oxygen, as does aerobic exercise. According to many of the Oriental systems, there exists in the air another element, variously called *prana, ch'i,* or *ki.* This is not a chemical element but a spiritual energy, the elemental life-force of the universe. It is believed that nothing survives without *prana,* that your vitality and health are primarily dependent upon its presence and its unobstructed flow throughout your body. (The Chinese system of acupuncture, for example, is based on removing blockages to the free circulation of *ch'i* by inserting thin metal needles at various points on the body.)

If you are practicing breathing exercises, it's helpful just to imagine this vital energy entering your body with each breath, and distributing itself all through you, from head to feet. Imagine that you are storing up life-energy with each deep breath you take. When you're sitting quietly you can certainly get along—that is, survive—on 5 or 6 quarts of air per minute, which is the dismal average today. But if you practice breathing more completely, so that you are taking in 10, 20, even 30 or 40 quarts per minute, what do you think the effects will be?

Remember that during strenuous physical exercise over 100 quarts per minute is possible, so doubling or

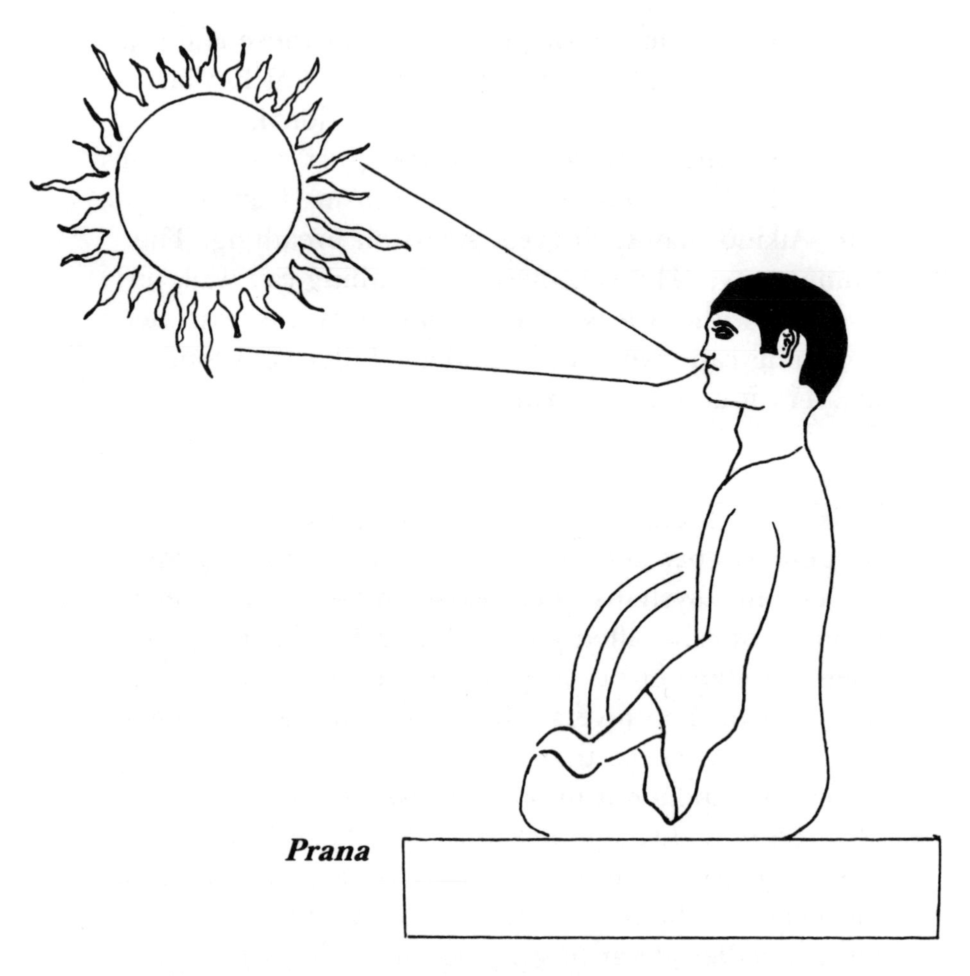

Prana

tripling your present intake is really not so much. You can double the air, double the oxygen, double the *prana.* The entire Yogic practice of Pranayama is based on this storing up of reserve *prana,* which gives the practitioner tremendous vitality, endurance, and just plain energy in general. Breathe on, Macduff!

These Oriental systems also lay great stress on inhaling *only through the nose.* Supposedly, *prana* cannot be as readily absorbed from the air in the mouth as in the nasal passages. Whether or not this is so, it *is* true that nature has brilliantly designed the nose, the nasal passages, and the sinuses to filter and catch impurities in the air we breathe—such as dust, excessive moisture, pieces of dirt, and so on. The nasal passages also warm up air that is too cold, and cool off air that is too hot. In general, the nasal system purifies the air you breathe and prepares it before it reaches the lungs.

The mouth is not equipped to do all this. As far as breathing is concerned, it was intended as an emergency channel only—for use when the nasal passages are blocked, or when a really great amount of air must be inhaled or exhaled in a very short time. When you're coming up for air after being underwater a long time, or when you're sick with a bad cold and your nose is stuffed up, or when you've gotten really out of breath sprinting 200 yards at absolutely top speed and are panting to catch your breath—at times like these, breathing through your mouth is natural. But the rest of the time, the nose is the organ nature designed for breathing.

Unfortunately, most people today are *mouth breathers* most of the time. This fact alone accounts for the high incidence of throat and respiratory infections—dust particles and bacteria enter through the mouth and infect either the throat or the lungs themselves. Those of you who are especially prone to colds and sore throats would do well to change to nose-breathing. I was a mouth-breather myself until several years ago, and I know.

Also, the low energy level of most people today may be due, at least in part, to the lack of *prana* caused by improper breathing. I can personally vouch for the fact that breathing through your nose while running long distances definitely improves your endurance. (And what is life but a long-distance run?) The effort required to change your breathing habits is not a small one—but it's worth it. Nose-breathers smell better too! (No pun intended!)

How do you go about learning (that is, relearning) to breathe through your nose?

1. The first thing is to completely clear your nostrils and upper nasal passages. You can do this in several ways:
   - Blow your nose really well, being sure to get both sides.
   - Gargle with *hot* salted water and wash your face, especially the nose and forehead, with *cold* water (the contrast of temperatures stimulates the flow of mucus). *Then* blow your nose.
   - Sniff a small amount of warm (not hot), lightly salted water up one nostril, then expel it by blowing. Do the same on the other side. This is painful at first try, but it works.
   - Breathe rapidly in and out, through the nose only. This will expel some very-hard-to-dislodge obstructions up there.
2. When you have succeeded in really clearing both nostrils, then practice Complete Breathing as I have described it. When you are comfortable with this practice, go on to the Alternate-Nostril Breathing Exercise (pp. 137–138).
3. Once you feel pretty secure doing breathing exercises through your nose while sitting or lying down, then start practicing nose-breathing while working, doing things around the house, walking—and work up to the point where you can maintain nose-breathing during a jog or slow run. This is much more difficult because you need to inhale and exhale a much greater volume of air, so your nasal passages have to be really clear and your lung action powerful.

   (During very strenuous exertion it's often a good idea to keep inhaling through your nose, but *exhale* through your mouth. This gets rid of the stale, used air as quickly as possible, while still retaining the advantages of nasal air filtration and the absorption of *prana.* Many people who put out a lot of energy, for one purpose or another, use some version of this technique: the karate shout, the "huh!" sound of the chain-gang worker, the shot-putter's yell. Any good strong exhale, using your stomach muscles to help it along, will serve most purposes: Breathe in through the nose—then out, hard, through the mouth. Try it the next time you have some really heavy work to do.)

4. An indispensable aid in keeping your nasal passages clear so that you can breathe through your nose is the plain old handkerchief. Carry one around with you and use it whenever you feel the slightest obstruction to your nose-breathing. Don't be embarrassed to blow your nose! The longer you maintain clear, free nose-breathing, the more comfortable you'll feel with it. Ultimately, a breath drawn in through the mouth alone will feel inadequate and lifeless to you. Then you won't have to *think* about it anymore—your natural "sense of breath" will have returned.

Rhythmicity of breath is another important factor. If you take up long-distance running or swimming, you'll soon discover that timing your breaths to your pace gives you much better endurance than just breathing haphazardly and irregularly. For example, if you run on a "6-count"—that is, inhale for three strides, exhale for three strides—and maintain that count over a mile run, you will tire much less easily than if you just breathed any old way. Try it and see. When you practice Complete Breathing, and any other breathing exercises, it's sometimes a good idea to observe a rhythm as well. For instance, inhale for 8, hold for 4, exhale for 8. Regularizing your breathing when practicing helps to regularize it in your daily life.

The point of paying so much attention to your breathing now is *to change your unconscious, habitual pattern* into a deeper, more complete, more regular, more natural, and more healthy one. Nobody wants to be thinking about their inhalations and exhalations for the whole waking day—and you don't have to. But it is necessary to become conscious of your breathing pattern now, so you can change it for the better; then it can become unconscious again.

Another advantage of making your breathing conscious is that this enables you to control your breathing at any time. When you are tense, anxious, fearful, suffering physical or emotional pain, or in any difficult, stressful situation, your breathing reflects this state. Usually it becomes more shallow, irregular, and high in the chest; some people actually stop breathing altogether when they get really frightened! At such times, if you concentrate on deepening, slowing, and regularizing your breathing, it will have an almost immediate therapeutic effect: your mind will become calmer and clearer, your body will relax and yet have more energy, you will feel tranquilized without chemicals, your fear and pain will be reduced, and you will be able to deal with the difficulty in a more positive way.

It is not important whether the breathing change actually has this effect directly, or whether the process of attending to yourself and your most vital life-function, before anything else, is the important thing (and the breathing just an outward sign of this). The fact is that natural, deep breathing and a relaxed, positive state of bodymind are pretty much the same thing. But you can know this only by doing it.

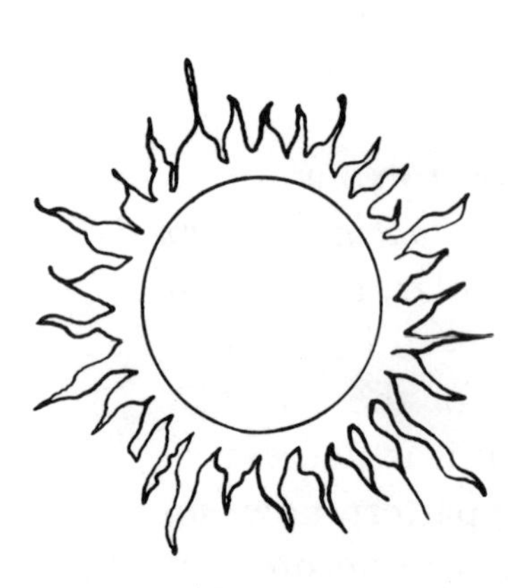

FLEXIBILITY AND RELAXATION

> Alive, a man is supple and yielding; in death, hard and stiff. All creatures and plants, alive, are supple and pliant, and dead, are withered and brittle. Therefore, to be hard and stiff is the way of death; to be supple and yielding is the way of life.
>
> LAO TZU

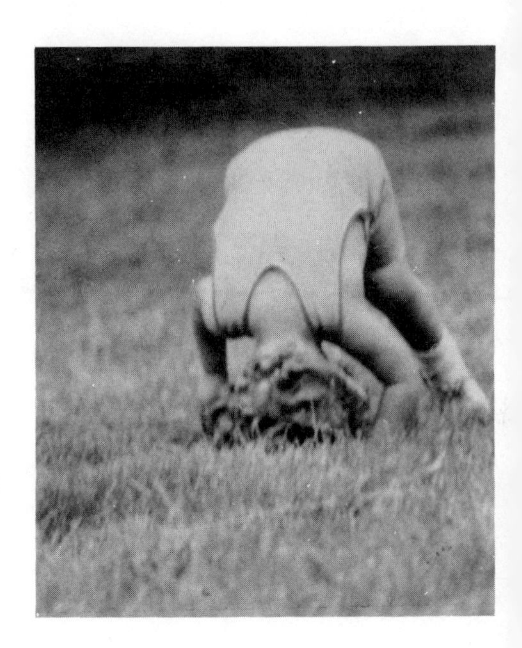

Several years ago I become aware of an imbalance in my physical development. My upper body was more muscular, more energetic, more identified-with, more "conscious" than my lower half. My shoulders, arms, and hands felt strong and competent; my hips, legs, and feet felt relatively weak, stiff, and unused. My roots, my contact with the earth, my foundations were not adequate to the structure above them.

At the same time I recognized a similar imbalance in my character and way of life. I was very competent, forceful, well-developed in all kinds of things that were a little "off the ground"—ideas and theories and impractical information (however impressive) and abstract subjects of all kinds. I was a good speaker with opinions on a wide variety of subjects, and was regarded as quite an influential person in my community. But as for the basic, down-to-earth root involvements of family, work, home, peace of mind, and the simple skills of living—in these I was neglectful, inept, and deficient. I was a top-heavy personality.

Over the years since I became aware of these things, I have worked at lowering my center of gravity—in the physical sense, by strengthening my legs and hips, using my lower body more, and being more conscious of my feet, ankles, and legs; while also learning to relax my upper body, breathe lower down, and so on. At the same time my character has altered, so that I am now less inclined toward abstract notions, ideas with no basis in the real world, theories, ideologies, unnatural values. I am more moved by the beauty and the power of life on this earth—by sexual love, by children, by wild animals and wilderness, by my family and my friends, by just plain living well. My body changes and my life changes turned out to be the same change. How could it have been otherwise?

One of the most common body difficulties people have is *lack of flexibility.* The most common inflexibility, and the one that is most damaging to your overall health, is inflexibility of the spine. We talked about the spine a little before. It's the communication route between the body and the brain. All information—sensory, kinesthetic (internal sense of movement), mental—travels along the spine, in the form of electrical impulses.

Almost everything you can think of involves the spine and requires proper functioning of the array of nerve cells comprising the spinal cord. All interaction between the inner world of your bodymind system and the outer world of everything else depends on the spine. For example, you touch a hot pan; nerve impulses travel from your fingers, up the spine to your brain, communicating this information. In the brain it is determined that this information refers to a situation of danger to you, the total organism. A new message is sent, again down the spinal cord, to the muscles of your arm and hand, making them contract in such a way as to withdraw your fingers from the hot surface as fast as possible. Your hand, you see, can't move of its own accord—it has to be instructed to do so by your brain (not necessarily your conscious brain, though, as in this case where the reaction is instinctual and dictated by the rear brain). But your brain can't *feel* anything by itself—it only acts on information received through the vast network of nerves. The vital link is the spine.

Most people today suffer from not being able to bend their spines forward, backwards, to either side, or in a twisting motion. This lack of flexibility may be caused by long-term tensions of certain back muscles that control the movement of the spine; or it may be due to structural problems of the bony spinal column itself. Lordosis (excessively curved spine) and scoliosis (crooked spine) are the two major types of this second, structural deformation. In either case, the stiffness of the spinal column interferes with normal functioning of the nervous system—and can have further unhealthy effects on virtually any part of your bodymind.

An example:

Next time you find yourself feeling a bit cold, try loosening up your spine with the four flexes that follow. You will be amazed at how much warmer this immediately makes you feel. Apparently stiffness of the spine slows down or even cuts off some of the nervous system communications, so that information regarding blood circulation to your extremities may be reduced, making you cold. Loosening up your spine restimulates the full flow of nervous system energy, body-brain communication is fully reestablished, blood is sent to the needy extremities, and you get warmer. Try it.

The point I made earlier, about the parallel nature and the interconnection of your body and your character, holds very true for the spine. Spinal inflexibility is usually associated with a basic inflexibility of character. We'll get back to this later. Right now, here are the four spinal flexes, which are not only good tests of your spine flexibility but also good exercises for improving it.

Spinal Flex One • Stand up straight, with your feet shoulder-width apart and slightly toed-in. Stretch your arms way up over your head while taking in a deep, slow breath.

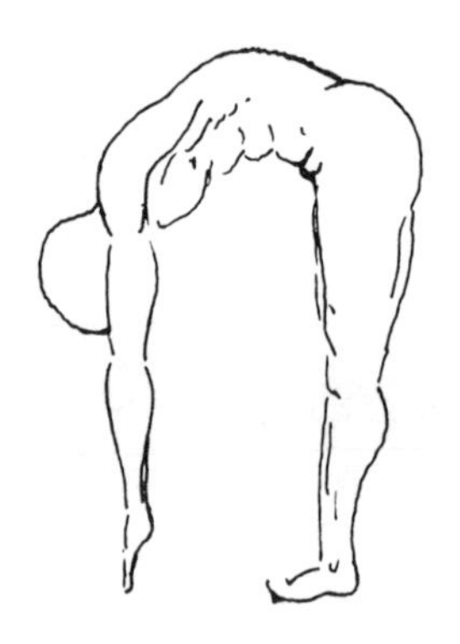

Exhale, letting your trunk bend forward until your hands reach the floor—*allow your knees to bend*—and let your head drop between your shoulders. Stay in this bent-over position, with a little weight resting on your hands (fingertips are okay if you can't bend over that far, or even leaning on a low chair or table), and relax. Try to curve your spine as much as possible, from the coccyx (base) to the back of your head. Tuck your head in, raise the middle of your back, and rotate your pelvis forward to increase the flex. Straighten your legs a little. Breathe deeply a half-dozen times in this position. Then slowly straighten up on the inhale, leaving your hands at your sides. Exhale and relax. This tests (and improves) the forward flexibility of the spine and stretches your back muscles and the hamstring muscles on the back of your legs.

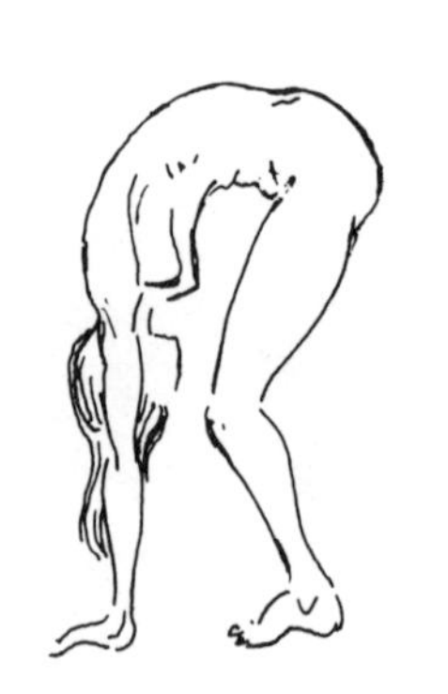

Variations:

1. When you're bent over as far as you can go on your own, have someone push gently but firmly on your upper back and the back of your head for extra stretch. Don't go into the pain range, but plenty of pressure is okay. Hold through a few breaths, then release.
2. While in the fully-flexed position, take the weight off your hands and bounce up and down a little, using gravity to stretch you even more. Shake your shoulders as you do this to keep the muscles completely relaxed. Let your arms and head dangle loosely, like a rag doll's.

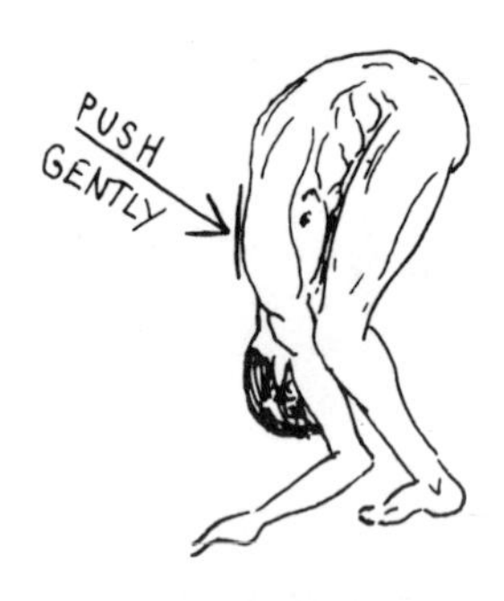

Spinal Flex One

Spinal Flex Two • Stand straight, with your feet a little wider apart than in #1. Inhale. Exhale and lean back, with your hands (palms or fists) on the small of your back. Lean back as far as you can comfortably; let your head roll back. If you're worried about your balance in this position, lean over the back of a couch or something else soft (a tall stool with some padding on it is good). Or have someone support the small of your back with

Spinal Flex Two

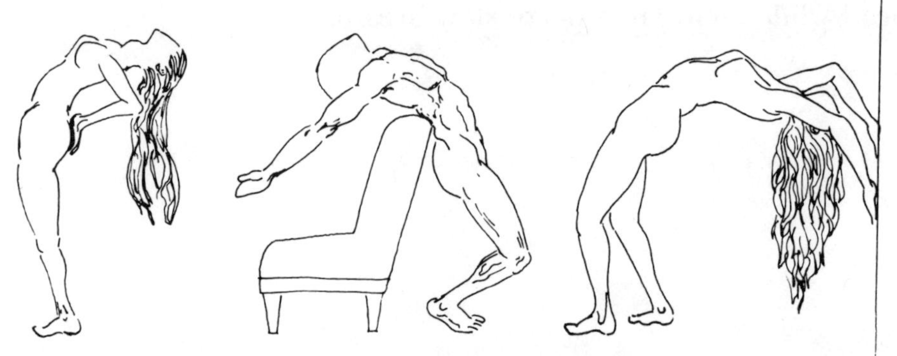

their arm. In these supported positions you can stretch your arms overhead as well, which will increase the pull on the upper part of your body. Hold the flexed position through several breaths, as relaxedly as possible. Rise slowly (don't turn sideways!) on an inhale; exhale and relax. This tests the backwards-arching flexibility of the spine, besides stretching muscles and tendons in the front of your thighs, hips, chest, shoulders, and neck.

Be sure to work on this flex very gradually, never going further than a strong pulling feeling. Keep your back muscles *completely relaxed* throughout—let gravity do all the work!

Variation:

Lean backwards and put your hands on a wall or doorway and "walk" them downwards as far as you can go comfortably, hold for a few breaths, then "walk" them up again.

Spinal Flex Three • Stand with your feet wide apart and your hands at your sides. Inhale. Exhale, leaning to the left, with your left hand on the outside of your left thigh for support. Stretch sideways as far as possible, toward your left foot, bringing your right hand overhead and to the left. Let your head drop toward the left shoulder as well. Be sure to keep both feet flat on the floor. Stretch as far as you can and relax into the position. Breathe there several times. Then straighten up while inhaling and drop your hands, exhale, relax. This one flexes your spine sideways. Repeat it to the right side.

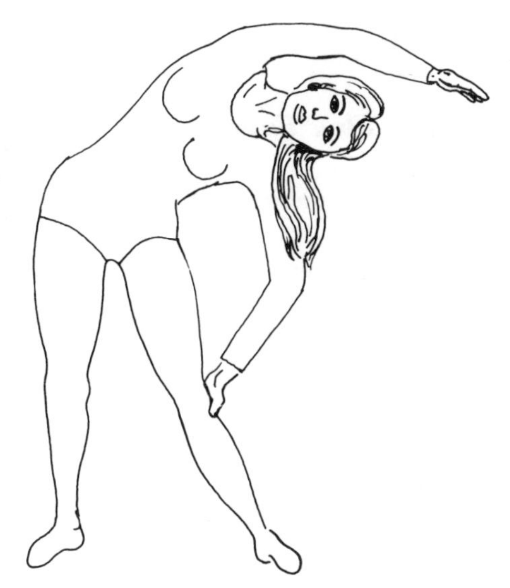

Spinal Flex Three

Variation:

Stand with your feet close together, about a foot and a half from a wall, facing sideways to the wall. Put both hands on the wall at about shoulder level. Now lean the middle of your body away from the wall as far as possible, keeping your hands and feet in position. This produces the same flex.

Spinal Flex Four • Stand with your feet wide apart and inhale, raising your arms out to the sides. Swing your whole trunk (hips to shoulders) alternately to the left and right, exhaling slightly on each turn. Allow your arms to dangle and swing freely as your body turns, so that they slap your back and shoulders at the end of each turn. Let yourself turn up onto the toes of your right foot while turning left, and left foot while turning right—but keep the other foot flat on the floor. Let your head turn simultaneously with your body. Your shoulders and head should turn quite a bit further than your hips—this flexes your spine in a twisting or "wringing" motion. Be sure to breathe out on each turn (helps you twist further); you can catch a short inhale as you twist back to the center.

You'll probably hear your back "cracking" on this flex, and maybe on the others as well. Don't be alarmed by this, it's a good sign! Repeat the turns to both sides on flex #4 several times, trying to "wring" your spine a little further each time.

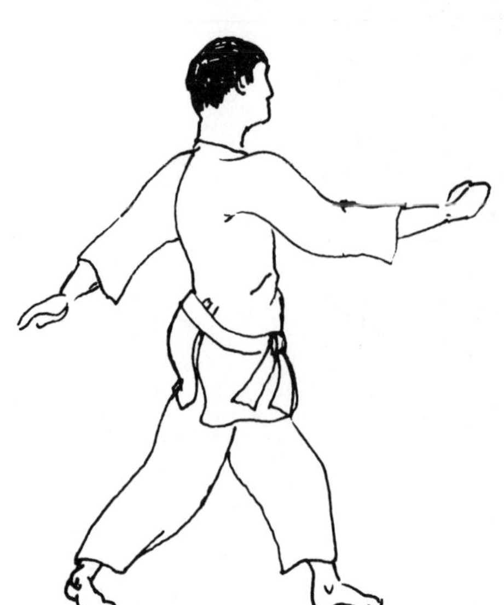

Spinal Flex Four

Variation:

Have someone stand behind you, bracing your feet with his or hers, to prevent them from overturning. Then have the person twist your shoulders around as far as they will go, while your hips and legs keep more or less the same position. This variation is good because you can relax your own back muscles completely while being twisted, since you don't have to use those muscles to power each turn.

These are the four main flexes of the spine. In a really healthy body they should be accomplished easily and without discomfort, with a large degree of bend in every one of the four directions. If this isn't the case with you—work on them!

As you test and practice spinal flexibility you will also notice other areas of tension, stiffness, or discomfort.

Right? Most people in our society are stiff and unbending over much of their bodies. The most "popular" areas of tenseness are the following:

1. ***The shoulder and back-of-neck muscles*** Usually tension here has been caused directly by some fear or anxiety (driving a car is the most common source of this tension). It's as if you were drawing your head in like a turtle, trying to protect your neck by raising your shoulders.
2. ***The eyes*** Tenseness in the eyes can be caused by straining to see, by wearing some kinds of glasses, and by mental strain. See Part III, Chapter Six, on the Bates Eye System.
3. ***The diaphragm and ribs*** Fear of deep inhalation or exhalation, which signifies fear of aggressive living or fear of letting go, is related to a stiff diaphragm and rib cage. Shallow breathers often have trouble learning Complete Breathing because of this tension. Young children don't have it.
4. ***The lower back*** This is a very common tension area. Stiffness here can be caused by overweight, sexual inhibitions (unconsciously pulling your genitals back and out of sight), and wrong posture—especially from sitting in soft chairs.
5. ***The pelvic region***—including the hip joints, the lower abdomen, and the buttocks. Tension here indicates a rigid, unhealthy separation of the upper and lower body and may reflect sexual inhibitions or deeper sexual problems such as impotence and frigidity. The lack of a full range of natural movements—running, squatting, kneeling, leaping, walking over varied terrain—also contributes a great deal to this kind of tension.
6. ***The ankles and feet*** Improper footwear, not enough barefoot walking and running, too much sitting and too little natural movement all serve to make your ankles and feet weak and stiff. This tension can affect the position of your pelvis and your spine (too much weight on the heels, for example, tends to rotate your pelvis backwards, producing overcurvature of the lower spine) and may ultimately contribute to disorders of the internal organs, the nervous, circulatory, and glandular systems, and even the sexual function. Weak arches, for example, fail to cushion the shock of walking, running, and landing on your feet after jumping (or even walking down stairs)—which may cause you headaches or even, as some have claimed, damage to the brain.

Take a few minutes now to check yourself out. Exam-

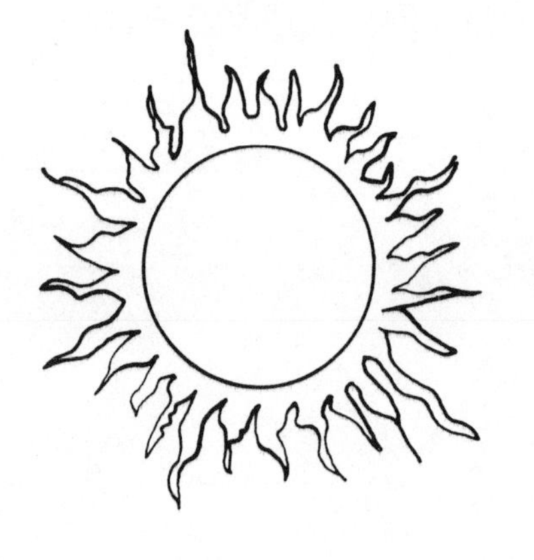

ine these major tension areas of the body and see what you find. You may come across other tensions as well, or parts of your body that just don't want to move freely and easily. I suggest even making a list of all your problem areas, so you can then proceed to work on them in a systematic and successful way.

Some tensions can be reduced—at least temporarily —by *massage.* This should be done gradually and firmly, preferably with some lubricating agent such as olive oil, hand cream, soapy water, or any lotion you like the feel and the smell of. Some parts of the body, like the feet and ankles, you can do pretty well yourself; others, like your shoulder muscles, are much better done by someone else. Massage of either kind is a delightful and very healthy experience. Do it often.

Finally, you should acquire the ability to relax away tension from any part of your body-and-mind just by turning your attention to it. You can gain the control to send the message of relaxation and positive, vital energy to any part of you, at will.

This may seem like a tall order, but you *can* cultivate the ability. Here's a way to begin: Lie down on a firm surface, with no restrictive clothing. Starting with your feet, and working all the way up to your scalp, systematically tense, and then relax, every single muscle in your body over which you have conscious control. This includes all the external-movement muscles (as opposed to the internal, organ muscles like the heart). Tense them one at a time, then relax them. Tensing first is easier, and establishes your control over the muscle's action; then relaxing the same muscle comes readily. You may find some muscles that are already in some kind of tensed state—if so, try to tense them even more (to establish control), then relax. Take your time, and go over your whole body. If you do this regularly (say, before going to sleep every night), it will soon give you a measure of control you never thought possible. You will be able to direct your attention to any place, and allow it to relax just by thinking. Incidentally, this systematic relaxation of the body from toes to head (be sure to include the face muscles, the stomach muscles, the neck, and the buttocks) is a great way to get to sleep if you're nervous or tense.

Why *is* it so important to relax and eliminate body tensions? Here are a few of the unhealthy results of tension:

1. It reduces your ability to move freely and easily.
2. It reduces your circulation and can even entirely cut off the flow of blood to the tensed area.
3. It desensitizes your body.
4. It can choke the functioning of your nervous system.
5. It can inhibit full, natural breathing.
6. It can prevent the necessary stimulation of the endocrine glands, the regulators of your body's inner chemistry.
7. It can produce a variety of other problems anywhere in your system.

> Tension . . . often the victim is a sensitive individual and has been through a particularly difficult period, perhaps involving the loss of a loved one or some similar crisis. This, of course, has contributed to a tension which can choke off circulation and prevent any organ from receiving proper nourishment. As a result, an ailment can develop anywhere in the body.
>
> LINDA CLARK, *Get Well Naturally*

It's not just major life problems that cause tension. The whole nature and design of our society, our technology, our civilization produces tension. For an example, let's take one of the most common activities in our society—driving a car. First of all, your hips and legs

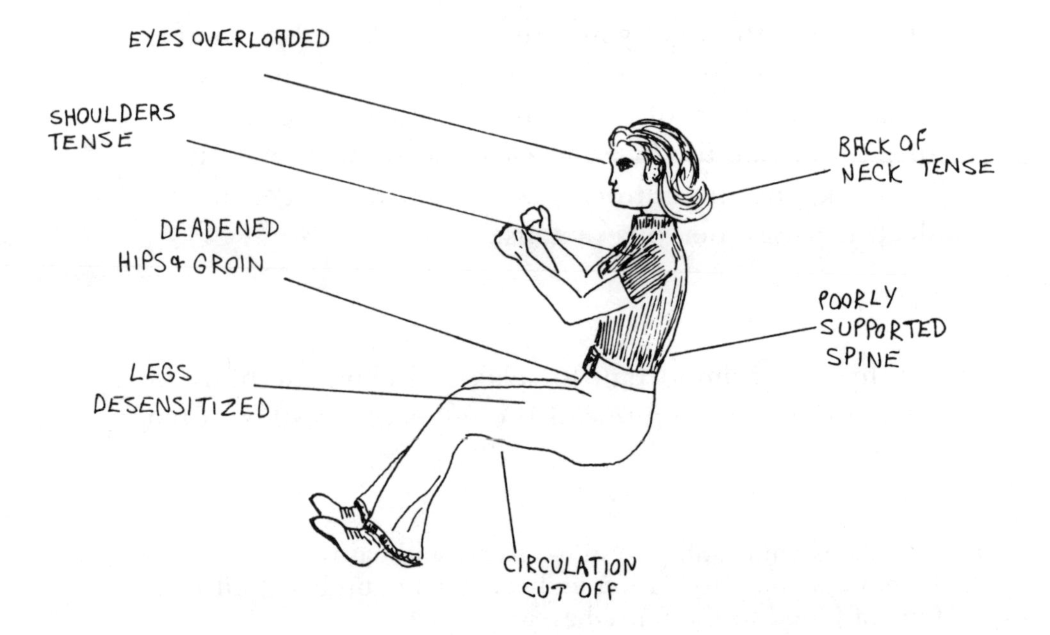

are barely used at all, so they become desensitized, almost numb. Your groin and pelvis are totally immobilized—there is only one position you keep them in for the entire time you are driving, and it's impossible to move them. Your whole lower body is deadened and stiff.

Second, your eyes and shoulder muscles are overloaded with responsibility. The smallest detail of movement, either of your eyes in watching the road, or of your arms in turning the wheel, spells the difference between life and death. Nervous energy floods the eyes and shoulders—and tension accumulates there. (Check your shoulder muscles and the back of your neck after your next long drive.)

Finally, there is the factor of the car seat. I have never been in or seen a car seat that allowed you to sit up straight in a balanced, centered, spine-straight posture—which is the only way you can sit without straining your back and spine. The car seat cuts off some circulation to your legs because of the pressure on your upper thighs. It makes you lean back so that the weight of your upper body falls somewhere at the middle or lower spine, rather than straight down through your hips. The car seat compels an incredibly unhealthy posture—but we all accept it and ignore the damage it does to us. Like sheep.

It's not only automobile driving, it's a thousand little elements of our daily lives—street noises, pressured work situations, emotional conflicts, sexual tensions, furniture you can't sit in with a living body, harsh artificial lighting, architecture designed with no concern for the people using it and living in it, polluted air and water, the bombardments of the so-called "entertainment" media and advertising; in fact, the whole unnatural environment that most of us are forced to live in. All these things, and more, contribute to the daily buildup of physical tensions and body rigidities. We don't pay attention to them, because no single thing is enough to harm you very much by itself. But the accumulation of outrages on the natural living body begins to make us stiff, insensitive, and immobile—like corpses—when we should be most full of energy, feeling, movement, and life.

Worst of all, physical tensions almost always correspond to certain negative psychological states—fear, depression, helplessness, frustration, loss of feeling, inability to communicate or to love. There is no separation between the mind and the body—we only act as if it were so! *Inflexibility of the body signifies inflexibility of the mind, of the heart, of the spirit.* A stiff, unbending body indicates the tendency to:

a) Compulsive behavior—you have to do something, no matter what other difficulties it may cause, no matter what the outcome.
b) Mechanical behavior—you move, work, act like a machine, taking no pleasure in what you do, having no feelings about it.

c) Blocked expression—you have strong feelings inside but you cannot let them out. The armor of your tension is too tight around you. It won't let the world in, won't let the real you out.
d) Lack of spontaneity—you rarely, if ever, act on an impulse, on a whim without knowing exactly why, just because you "feel like it." Children are spontaneous in most of their behavior. But the rigid, unhappy, compulsive adults of our society could use a lot more of such childishness!

What *is* tension anyway? *Tension is a bodily response to a fear or threat you cannot really deal with.* Normally, when you are faced with something you're afraid of, you either *fight* against it in some fashion, taking direct, aggressive action; or you run away, you *escape* from it, taking a negative action for survival's sake, but an action nonetheless. Two choices—either you deal with a problem directly or you deal with it by escaping. But when, for any number of reasons, you *can't* choose between "fight or flight," or your fear is so great that you can't manage to *do* either, then your body stiffens, goes rigid, becomes "dead." It's as if, on an animal level, you were trying to fool a predator into thinking you're not a living thing. Sometimes rabbits and deer will panic and freeze like this in the lights of an oncoming car on the highway. It's an inappropriate, ineffective, and often deadly response to make—for man as much as for the rabbit.

Relaxed, flexible, energetic movement is always the best way to deal with a difficulty. Take falling, for example. Most adults, when they trip over something or lose their balance, immediately stiffen up—and hit the ground like a block of ice, or the proverbial "ton of bricks." Even a minor fall usually produces some injury—bruises at least, often broken bones or torn muscles and strained ligaments, and worse.

But look at the way a three-year-old child falls: body relaxed and supple, no tension stiffening the muscles and making the structure rigid. The child hits the ground softly, collapses, rolls, absorbs the impact of the fall—and gets up right away, usually laughing. It's enjoyable to fall that way, it's a little joke gravity plays on your body, a brief return to proneness during the day's verticality. Little kids fall like this *dozens* of times every day and think nothing of it—and remember they're falling from their own full height, just as you and I do. The average rigid, fearful adult would be in the hospital after the first five falls. Take a lesson from children!

It is possible to be *too* flexible, to have not enough control over your movements, your emotions, thoughts, and actions. This condition is seen in the body as an excessive looseness, a rag-doll appearance. In the mind it takes the form of impulsiveness—you do things, even dangerous or hostile things, because you "just can't help yourself." The most extreme form of this is a kind of schizophrenic state, in which you feel that impressions, feelings, forces, events move through you without any filtering-out mechanism. You feel subject to all kinds of influences but are powerless to resist them or make sense of them or integrate them into your own personality. The world rules you completely and you have no control.

So these are the two extremes: on the one hand, rigidity, tension, immobility, armoring, loss of feeling, fear, and much too strict and uncompromising control over everything; on the other hand, super-looseness, lack of control, no fixed sense of yourself, no self-defense, just forces and actions without any meaning. Most people in our society suffer more from too much tension than from too much looseness. But sometimes the schizophrenic overflexibility appears in someone who has been tightly bound up in himself or herself for a long time and finally "breaks out." This person may then go all the way to the opposite extreme, in a nervous breakdown, a freak-out, a spell of madness.

Health is a balance between the two extremes, a dynamic balance in which you are more controlled at some times, more spontaneous at others. But being stiff and rigid is never appropriate—while you're alive! You learn your own balance through free and flexible movement. Get back your natural mobility and you can enjoy the spontaneity of the child *and* the true self-control of the healthy adult. But you can't learn to follow your body's needs while your body is blocked, choked off, and desensitized by tensions—just as you can't get very far in knowing your own life needs if your growth is frozen by fears, worries, inhibitions, and rigidities of thought and feeling. The antidote to tension is one thing—*relaxation.*

I realize that it's very easy for me to tell you to relax, but a lot harder for you to actually do it. As a first step, why not just give yourself some time every day just to *be* —without any pressure to *do* anything or produce anything. Just let yourself be! This can be a time of mental *and* physical relaxation. Become sensitive to yourself. You might want to move around, you might want to sit still and think of nothing, you might want to take a walk or soak in a hot tub or massage your feet or take some time and slowly stretch out all your muscles. Give yourself what you need! But it will probably be better to do it alone, and without using any outside mechanism such as television, liquor, grass, pills, magazines, or anything else. This is because you want to give up, eliminate, *unlearn* your tensions and rigidities—not substitute something a little less painful in their place. The less outside stimulation you get, the more you will be able to really relax during these times. Just dig yourself for a while —and learn a little more about your body character. The two keys to health, two really magical keys, are flexibility and relaxation. Cultivate them, and see.

We'll finish the chapter with two relaxation practices —one is active, the other passive. Both are good to do when you're uptight.

Active Relaxation • Starting with your hands, wrists, and arms, *shake* your whole body. After the arms, do your feet and your legs—one at a time. Really shake them, long, hard, and good! Then shake your head, neck, and shoulders—bend forward at the waist (knees bent), let your head hang and your arms dangle, and shake your shoulders and head up and down, and from side to side. From this position, start shaking your legs in a quick, bouncing motion (both legs together). Stand up as you keep bouncing from the legs. Get your hips going in time with your legs, in a rapid, sexy motion. Finally you should be standing, knees bent, upper body relaxed, and every part of you shaking and vibrating together. Let your body go however it wants to. Feel the rhythm of your own flesh, all of it moving and shaking and feeling alive. Do this as long as you feel like it, then stop. Feels good, doesn't it?

Passive Relaxation • Lie down on your back on a firm surface—a soft mattress is no good. Bring your knees up and tie them together with a belt, a cloth, or a short piece of rope. (The tying makes sure that you won't have to use any leg muscles to keep the knees up and together.) Keep your feet on the floor. Cross your arms over your chest—if they'll stay crossed without your holding them there, fine; if not, lay them flat on the floor. Put something under your head to raise it an inch or two off the floor—but not as high as a regular pillow. In this position your entire spine should be straight and flush with the ground. If it's not, adjust your position until it is. If you have an overarched lower back, for example, so that the small of your back is still off the ground, then raise your legs by putting them up on a

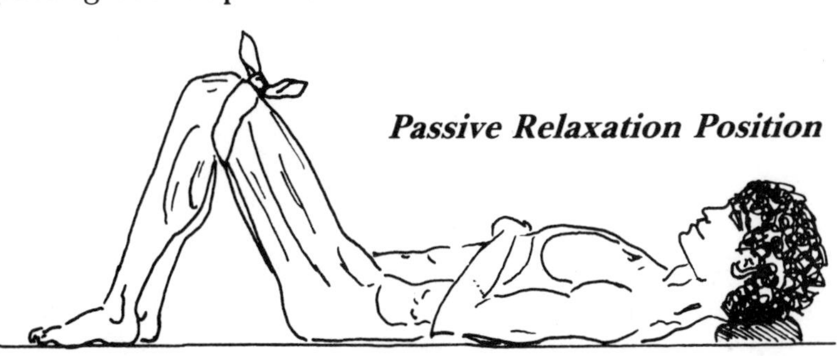

Passive Relaxation Position

chair or on a low table that gives you the right angle so that your lower spine lies flat on the floor. If you have the opposite problem, where the small of your back is on the ground but your coccyx bone is not, then you should lower your knees, by straightening your legs out, until the right angle is reached. Adjust your head, shoulders, and middle back in the same way. When your spine is straight and flush with the floor, close your eyes. Breathe deeply. This is a perfect relaxation position. You need absolutely no muscular effort anywhere in your body to maintain this position!

Slowly and systematically go over your whole body and release the tension from every part of it. Use your imagination on stubborn problem areas—like this: Pretend you are an empty suit of clothes, lying on the floor. Imagine the creases in the back of the jacket being slowly pulled from the bottom and the sides until they flatten out. The "creases," of course, are chronic tensions of back muscles, but imagining them as creases in a jacket helps you to relax them away. Take plenty of time in this position, and be sure to pay attention to every area of your body.

As your body relaxes and straightens out, let your mind do the same thing. Don't hurry, don't think of anything in particular, don't even *try* to relax those tense muscles so much—just *let* them relax. Let your own thoughts and feelings come and go. Let yourself just lie there, peacefully, untroubled, breathing deeply and evenly. Let any worries, problems, or fears you may have fall away from you in these quiet minutes. Let the world and its obligations, trials, and problems wait for *you.* You need this time to restore your inner balance, to be still and silent and free from fear. Let nothing matter—for a little while. Allow your mind to clear, allow your body to relax, allow yourself to be. Amen.

HARA (THE CENTER)

Stand up, with your feet slightly apart and your weight distributed evenly between the heel and the ball of each foot. Bend your knees slightly. Keeping your spine straight—and vertical—relax all the muscles of your upper body. Relax chest, shoulders, face, neck, arms, and back. Breathe slowly and evenly, from the belly. Keep your eyes closed.

Feel the whole weight of your upper body *sinking* down—although your spine remains erect. Let this weight settle in your lower abdomen, just below the navel. Feel the firm structure of your feet, legs, and hips *supporting* your relaxed and balanced upper body. Move a little from side to side, forward and back, twisting, gently shaking yourself, until you really feel *centered* at that place below the navel.

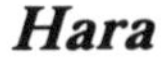

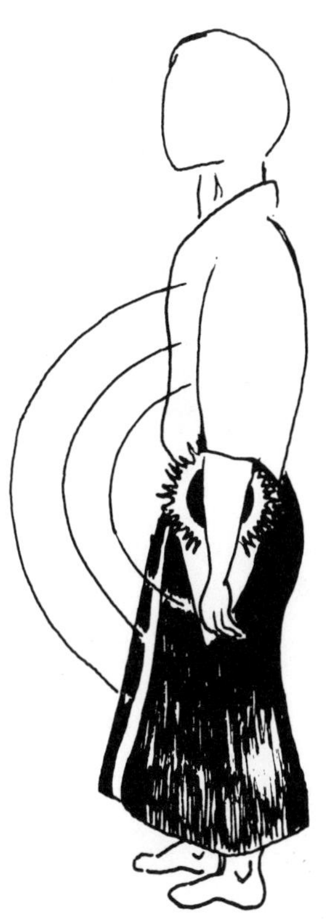

Concentrate your attention at this place. Keep relaxed, continue your deep breathing, and feel this area in your lower abdomen as your balance point. Now imagine that this place is the source of all your natural energies. Imagine a warm force spreading from here through your whole body, reaching your scalp, your toes, your fingertips.

When you feel like moving, open your eyes and go back to your normal activity. But try to keep the deep breathing, maintain the relaxed yet upright posture, and remember this center and the force that flows from it.

This is *Hara.* Physically, it *is* the balance point—the center of gravity for the whole upper body. This means that when your upper half is relaxed and straight (not tensed up or imbalanced in any direction), it acts as if the whole weight of it were concentrated at that one spot, in the lower abdomen below the navel.

In the Orient, Hara is also believed to be that one place where the body and the spirit intersect. The physical laws of the observable universe (like gravity) and the spiritual laws of man's inmost being are said to coincide in Hara. If your head is the center of thinking, consciousness, and rationality, then Hara is the center of Nature within you. It is the seat of the earth-forces, the instinctive, the root and source of your living energy. Remember in Part One we discussed the Paleolithic and the Rational? Your brain is the Rational center; Hara, the point in your lower abdomen, is the Paleolithic center.

We stand between earth and heaven, between pure Nature and pure Mind, between the physical and the ethereal. A healthy human life is a magnificent balance that integrates these two aspects into one whole being. But modern man has no balance. Mostly, he is all up and no down—all mind and thought, not enough legs and living. We reach out for the stars, we send men to the moon, we advance in science and technology and all the products of the mind. But the earth itself, the source of our life, the base, the root from which we grew—and from which we still must draw our only sustenance—this earth is in bad trouble, scarred, polluted, covered with concrete and the inorganic wastes of our ecologically corrupt way of life.

The Hara, the lower center, is your trust of Nature within you. It's your identification with everything that lives. It's the source of all vitality and natural energy. But most of us are out of touch with it. We do not feel it, we do not even believe in its existence. Like an uprooted plant that loses its connection with the earth, we only shrivel and stiffen, and then die. It need not be that way. Reestablish the Hara, and great Nature moves

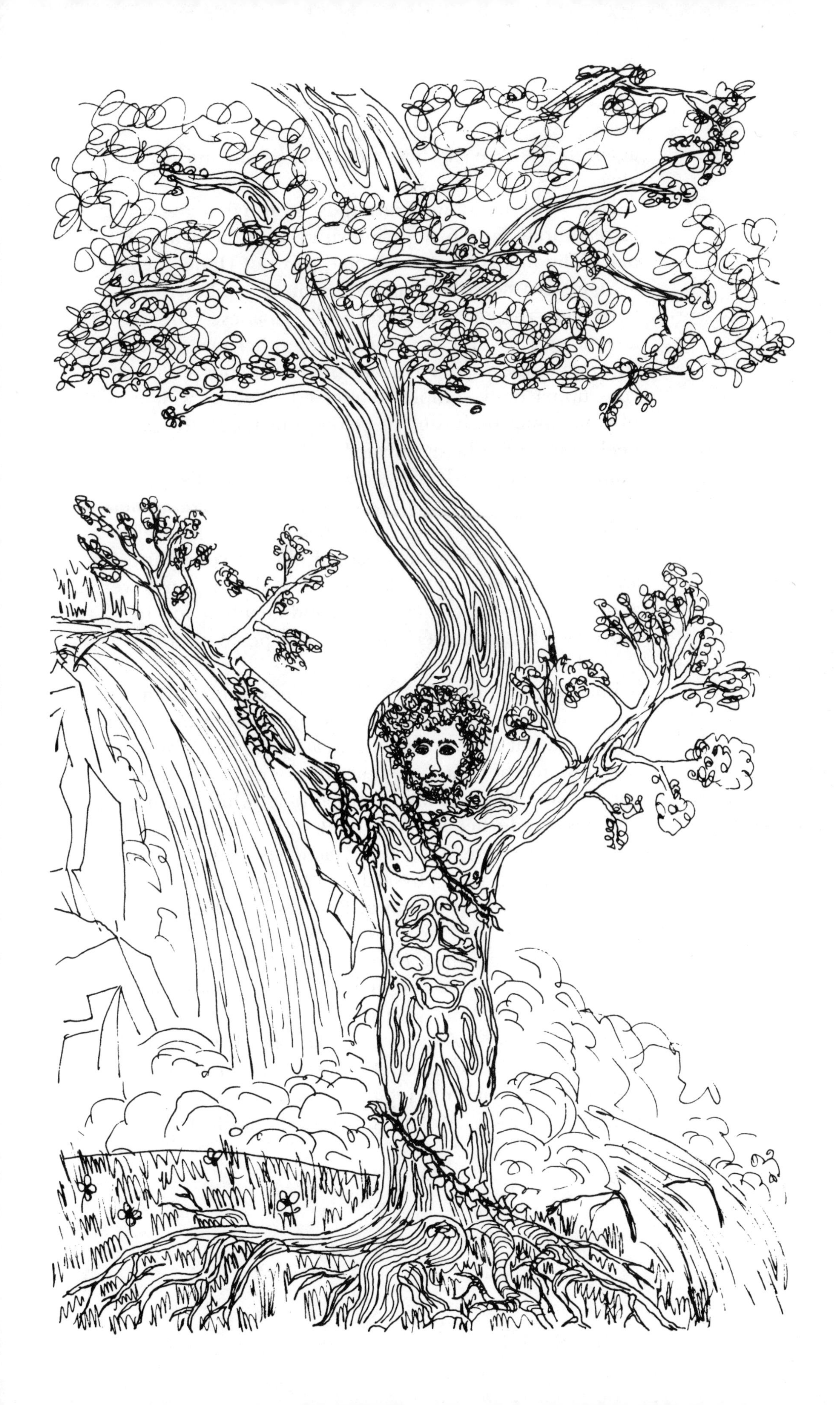

again in you. We can become whole again, and truly alive.

How? The mind and Hara must stop fighting—and instead unite, in a living triumvirate with the heart of man. The first step is to become *aware* of Hara:

Stand as I described before, or sit on a pillow with your legs crossed or on your heels, Japanese-style. (Use a chair only if you can't manage the other two.) Keep your spine erect, your neck aligned with your spine, and your upper body completely relaxed. Feel the weight of your upper body sink to below your navel, to Hara. Feel your breath being inhaled and concentrated at the same spot—then exhaled, slowly, from there also. Feel that you actually *are* that place, that you are *located* there rather than in your head, your chest, or anywhere else. Feel the strength in your legs and hips, in your buttocks and the small of your back, and especially in your lower abdomen, *supporting* your weight and enabling you to move swiftly and powerfully from this position, if you should so choose.

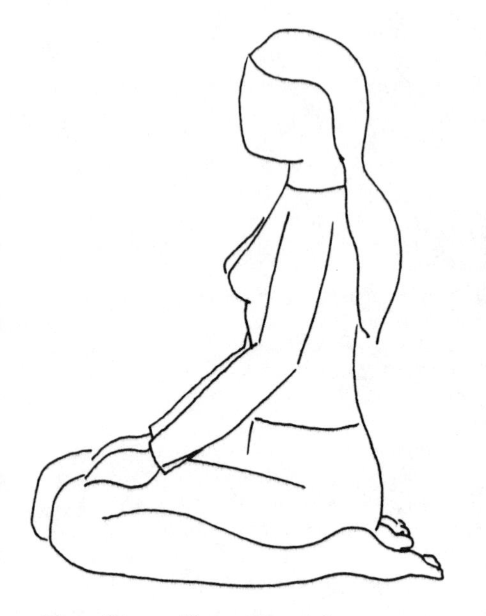

Zen Kneeling Position

Put your *mind* into Hara. This is the essential thing. It means not only thinking *about* the one spot in the lower abdomen, but almost thinking *from* there. You can practice this anywhere and anytime—every morning after you get up, while talking on the phone, while waiting on lines—and whenever you think of it. You will notice very soon the benefits of this practice to your posture, your breathing, your physical well-being, and, most importantly, your state of mind. But this is just the first step.

Next, practice *keeping Hara*—that is, keeping yourself centered in the lower abdomen, with your upper body relaxed and erect and your mind concentrated below your navel, *while moving.* Practice keeping Hara through the most simple and natural movements—first walking, then turning, spinning, jogging, running, squatting, kneeling, jumping. Moving this way should feel quite different from the ways you have moved before—more effortless, more coordinated, and more enjoyable!

If you can maintain your *breathing* from the belly as well as your concentration, you'll find that your stamina is increased considerably. You'll get tired less easily, and recover faster. Being centered in Hara is being like a child: no straining, no upward-pulling tensions, no overload of the mind. Yet life is full and everything gets done. Try it and see.

The first step was essentially a static body-meditation—sinking your weight to Hara and concentrating your attention there. The second step was a dynamic meditation-in-motion—keeping your center while walking, turning, moving about. The third step is the integration of Hara *in daily life.*

This requires that you practice the first two steps over a period of weeks and months until you become *rooted* in your legs and *centered* in your belly, so that you move from there, breathe from there, and *live* there.

When you reach that point you won't have to *think* about Hara, you won't have to consciously maintain it as your balance center. You will have regained a certain instinctual life-sense, the natural balance sustained *from below*—both physically and psychologically. How much better to feel balanced and supported by the earth, by your legs and hips, than pulled up by your mind, "hung up" on tensed shoulders and a tight back! And this instinctual earth-balance will be constantly correcting and readjusting itself, unconsciously and *without effort.* When you reach this point, your health—physical/mental/emotional, for they are all one—will be unshakable.

Maybe this all sounds too abstract and you want some proof. Who says Hara is the center? How can you be sure it works? Okay. Try this test, with a friend to help you:

Stand up with your feet a little apart. Tense your whole body, including the legs and back—but especially the chest, shoulders, neck, and arms. Swell out your chest—make yourself look strong like the muscle men of the magazines. Take your energy upwards, into your chest and head; concentrate your attention up there, identify yourself there. Have your friend push you, slowly and gently, at one shoulder, from the front.

You can easily be pushed off-balance, even toppled, right? *Now* relax your upper body, sink everything into your lower half (from the waist down)—into your belly, your hips, your legs, your feet. Breathe deeply and low down. Think down. Concentrate yourself below the navel, at Hara. Relax and keep your awareness there. Ask your friend to push you again, in the same way, slowly and gently. What happens?

You have become much harder to move, you keep your balance more easily, you don't even have to try to resist—right? This is centering in Hara.

Here's another way to verify what I've been saying: Look around you, at the people you work with, travel with, encounter on the street, live with. Observe their posture and their movement. You'll see mainly two things—*overtension* and *collapse.* People in a state of overtension are hunched up, tight, stiff, straining upwards against gravity. People in a state of collapse are more than relaxed—they're slouched, sagging, pulled down by gravity in bent and curved postures, defeated. These are the two extremes, and they're both unhealthy. Most people alternate between the two; they "get themselves up" for something (like work, a date, a performance) but it doesn't last, and pretty soon they're feeling "down" again.

The physical state of overtension corresponds to an

emotional-mental state of fear and anxiety and over-striving. The physical state of collapse corresponds to despair, weakness of character, oversusceptibility, aimlessness. Look at people carefully and you'll see what I mean.

Here and there you may see a really healthy, balanced person. You can tell this person by his or her posture, and by other things as well: speech, manner, energy, the kind of feelings you get from his or her presence. If you look at the posture, you'll notice neither the upwards-pulling tension nor the downwards-dragging slackness. Instead, you get the impression of a unified, balanced whole—the body erect, upright, vertical, yet relaxed, supple, and mobile. In a word, *centered.*

Observing such a person, you'll note the easy strength of the hips, legs, and abdomen—providing movement, grace, balance, and control. You'll also notice the balanced character, with neither the tendency to anxiety, fear, anger, or arrogance (the excessively upwards character), nor the tendency to depression, pessimism, despair, or dependency (the excessively downwards character). This unified balance is health of the whole bodymind.

The person who lives in Hara is in touch with the forces of Nature that are within us. He or she remains healthy, and does not lose that inner balance even in the most difficult, dangerous, or disordered situations. You can become centered in Hara also!

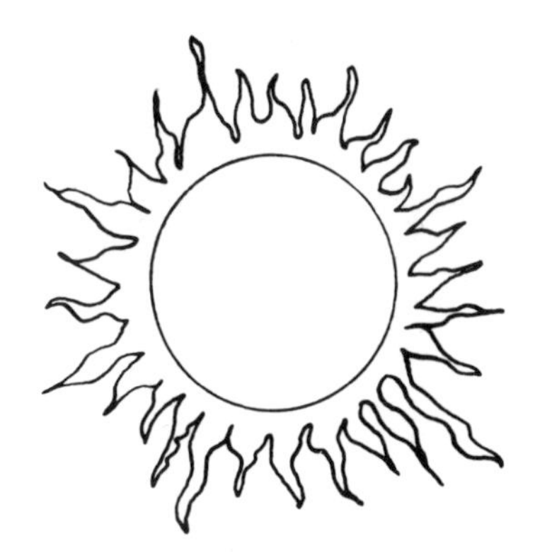

Practice breathing, practice right sitting, practice letting-go of tensions. Letting go of tensions is letting go of the mind's overpowering hold on your life. It's loosening the death-grip that fears, anxieties, guilt, regrets, images, ideas, unnecessary and unnatural needs have on your simple need to live. Letting your shoulders drop, and letting strength rise from Hara, is the same as letting all those ideas and mental obstructions go—and letting Nature rise, and flow in you. Nature heals, vitalizes, makes things grow. Hara is Nature in you—it has only to be uncovered and realized. The Zen master Hayashi, when asked how one should go about becoming a master of Hara, replied, "Just by letting the master who is in us come out."

All natural actions, especially those that come from your hips and legs, help to center you in Hara. Running is a good example—but you should run easily and gracefully and without straining. Be aware only of your feet, your legs, your hips, your breathing, the ground, your whole bodymind and your surroundings—anything else is extraneous. Almost all the work of running is done by the lower body, but still some people run from their heads. They keep themselves "located" in the chest and arms and face, barely feeling their feet and legs at all! I know—I used to be one of them. That kind of tense, anxious running won't do you half as much good as the relaxed, centered kind.

A simple thing like tying your shoelaces or picking up something from the floor can be an occasion to practice centering. Don't bend over stiffly from the waist, destroying your balance and losing Hara. Instead, as I described in Part I, kneel into a crouch with one foot flat and the other on the ball, keeping your spine straight and maintaining your center. How much more graceful, more natural, more powerful this is! Do it in front of a mirror and see.

Probably you've experienced the sensation of having a warm (or hot) head and cold feet. This is a sign of "upwardness"—the circulation of your blood is not balanced properly throughout your body. Too much going to the head, too little to the legs. Too much thinking, not enough walking! Move more, breathe lower, practice keeping Hara—and after a while you may get to the point where you have warm feet and a cool head. As the Chinese say, this is the most desirable of conditions!

Moving from the hips is another very good way of getting centered in the lower abdomen. What is "moving from the hips"? Very simple. Get up now and go to the window, and open it. Okay, how did you do it? Probably you began the action with your hands, or your head, right? That's because you *identify* most with those parts of you. But it made your movement out of balance, somewhat weak, and probably less than beautiful.

Now this time get up and repeat the action—but as if the "I" who is going to open that window is located in your hips. Start the movement with your hips. Let your legs, arms, hands, eyes, head, all do their jobs—but let the center lead! Notice any difference?

Moving from the hips *unifies* the power of your whole bodymind instead of dividing it into upper and lower, left and right, legs and head, and so on. This is why all the Oriental fighting arts, such as Karate, Aikido, and Kung Fu (see Part Three) teach that the power for *all* actions—whether of the feet, hands, head, or whole body—must come from the region of the hips.

Breaking bricks, boards, cinder blocks and such things with the hands or feet is neither very mysterious nor even very difficult for someone who has trained in any of the arts that understand and apply this basic principle of Hara. With the power of one arm alone it is impossible to break a brick. Obviously. But imagine dropping a 150-pound boulder in such a way that the weight of the stone landed at one small point, squarely in the middle of the brick. That would break the brick easily, wouldn't it? If a 150-pound man uses his whole body as one unit, moves from the center, and uses a relatively hard surface (such as the knuckles or the hand edge) for the impact point of himself-as-the-stone, then it's not hard to understand that the brick will break in this case too. *Moving from the center is the secret of great power!*

The Japanese call this power *ki;* the Chinese call it *ch'i;* the Hindus call it *prana.* It has many other names. It is said to accumulate in the lower abdomen and spread from there to all the limbs and organs of the body, as a life-energy or internal "spirit of vitality." The ways to cultivate this inner power are all the ways I have been telling you about:

1. deep abdominal and complete breathing
2. relaxation—not collapse
3. suppleness and flexibility, of body and of character
4. natural movement and closeness to nature
5. centralization in Hara
6. clarity and calmness of mind
7. a spirit of loving protection for all things

Ki is not a mysterious force, not something supernatural or occult or other-worldly. We see evidence of it all the time—children have it, people when they're really laughing have it, anytime you feel good you've got it. Incidents of a 100-pound woman lifting up the front of a 3000-pound car when her child is caught under it—that's ki too. Actually we could not live at all without at least some of it. Ki is life-energy.

But most of us obstruct the free flow of ki. This obstructing makes us sick, unhappy, and limited in our possibilities for living. Being tense, imbalanced, fearful, sedentary, and overcivilized blocks the stream within. By reopening the lower center we are allowing ki to flow in us again—as it flows already in the tree, the deer, the leopard, and the child.

Here's the simplest and easiest way of all to practice Hara: spend some time (five minutes is fine to start) *moving without using your arms.* Try sitting, kneeling, lying down and getting up, anything at all—but let your arms hang from your shoulders like a rag doll's. Don't use them for support, or even for balance. Let all the work be done by your legs, hips, back, stomach, and belly. You'll be in for a surprise!

Try it first on a rug, a mat, a lawn, in a field, or on any *soft* surface—because you'll probably fall around a bit. Try lying down flat on your back, pausing, then rising to standing position again, all without using hands, shoulders, or arms. Interesting, eh? Then try the same thing from lying on your stomach. Try sitting cross-legged (don't use your hands to adjust your feet!) and then get up. Try kneeling. Try all sorts of things with your body, minus your arms.

It may seem hard at first, you may feel clumsy or strange. But in another way it's a delightful feeling, isn't it? This practice makes you aware of how much unconscious tension and imbalanced energy we keep in our upper bodies all the time. (It's just like the residual volume of air kept in the lungs of shallow breathers who can't exhale enough.) This is a great way to relax *in movement.* Try it.

Becoming centralized in your lower abdomen, though,

> . . . is a technique, a device, a form of training or discipline, not an end in itself. It has as its final aim the achievement of total coordination and harmony of mind and body, of man and men, of man and his environment (now expanded to include the whole universe).
>
> WESTBROOK AND RATTI, *Aikido and the Dynamic Sphere*

Hara is the balance point of the living organism. Find it in yourself!

SEX, AND LOVE

Relax for a minute and think honestly about your sex life. (Be your own psychiatrist!) How would you describe it? Is sex a free and open source of pleasure for you, uninhibited and joyful? (Always? Sometimes? Never?) Is your sex life free from "outside" pressures and anxieties? Is your sexual activity, whatever it is, the kind you really desire—and of the frequency you desire? (Yes? No? Sort of?) Would you say that your sexual experiences are completely satisfying, affording you a total release of biopsychic (bodymind) energy? Be honest with yourself. And if your sex life isn't satisfying, *why isn't it?*

The bodymind factors I've been talking about up to now—movement, breathing, flexibility, relaxation, centeredness—are all vitally important for a healthy sex life. Tension and weakness of the hips, abdomen, buttocks, and thighs, for example, can reduce the feeling and the energy of your sexual activity. Not breathing in or out fully also reduces your sensation, inhibits your full freedom of movement, and deprives you of life-energy, of which sex-energy is a particular form. (Sighing, moaning, crying, laughing, all require full breathing. Have you sighed, moaned, or guffawed lately?) Aerobic exercise gives you the cardiovascular endurance for the most vigorous lovemaking. And becoming centered in Hara means that you come to sex, and love, as a whole person, a unified bodymind.

Many people mistakenly seek solutions to their sexual and emotional difficulties by attempting to cure one part rather than the whole person. The psychiatric approach, for example, is premised on the idea that the *mind* alone is the source of all sexual disorders. The original "psychic" cause for a pattern of impotency or frigidity is sought in an exclusively mental context (psychotherapy or psychoanalysis). On the other hand, there are many who attempt simply to retrain the *body* to its normal sexual functioning while ignoring any psychological roots of the disorder. The popularization of many of the Masters and Johnson techniques (such as the Seamans "squeeze" technique for premature ejaculators) has led to their misuse; few people appreciate the extensive counseling, psychiatric investigation, and careful preparation of an emotionally unthreatening context that must form the base of this sex therapy before the techniques themselves are ever employed.

The point is, no approach can be successful unless it deals with the whole person. *There is no disorder that exists only in the mind, or only in the body.* It may be true that most sexual dysfunctions originate with some psychic event—the punishment or rejection or humiliation of sexual feelings, for example. On the other hand, all neuroses and psychoses and hangups and depressions and failures, and all manner of "mental" or "emotional" disturbances, are also rooted in the body. They are located somewhere in the physical system, as pain, or tension, or weakness, or insensitivity, or imbalanced structure, or organ malfunction, or blocked energy flow. Any "cure" that deals with only the body *or* the mind, and ignores the other, cannot work.

Example One:

A "frigid" woman, who is not actually frigid in the sense of cold or unfeeling but is unable to reach orgasm. As a child she was caught masturbating by her parents and acquired a deep sense of guilt about sexual feelings. She developed the unconscious habit of tensing her abdomen and holding her breath as she came close to orgasm, thus cutting off the pleasurable feelings and punishing herself for sexual activity. Years later, although her parents have died and she has been able to recall the original trauma on a psychiatrist's couch, the problem remains. Why? Because, although the psychic cause *has* been eliminated, the negative body pattern of tensing and not breathing on the brink of orgasm remains—and makes the woman nonorgasmic. Dealing only with her psychological history does not constitute a complete or effective therapy.

Example Two:

An impotent man who has gradually lost his sexual potency over a six-month period since he was laid off from his job, and has been unable to find new work. His wife has had to take a part-time job, although she never worked before. He is demoralized, and his sexual performance shows it. He buys a paperback that claims to give the inside story on a famous and expensive form of sex therapy that the reader can practice at home. Skipping the theoretical chapters, he reads only the part that tells how to retrain himself to "get it up" and keep it up. Over the weekend he and his wife follow the directions and have several reasonably good sex experiences. But Monday several bills arrive that he hasn't the money to pay, and his job-hunting is fruitless. That night he tries to make love again, but his impotence recurs. The purely physical "cure" did not last.

There is no such thing as a "sexual" disorder that exists by itself in an otherwise completely healthy person. The sexual dysfunction is only one symptom, a *manifestation of trouble in the whole bodymind.* An impotent man is not just impotent sexually—he is impotent sexually because he is impotent in life, because he *feels* impotent (that is, "not powerful") either physically, socially, economically, emotionally, or some other way. Stated simply, the disease itself is a feeling of powerlessness, of blocked or reduced energy; the inability to get or maintain an erection is just one (very noticeable and highly distressing) symptom.

Every problem of this sort should be recognized as a

cycle involving many areas of the bodymind at once—some of which are quite observable and seem more easily accessible to treatment, and some of which are quite hidden, often unrecognized. It is not so important which particular part of the cycle is dealt with first in treatment (for example, the sexual failure, or the feelings of inadequacy and inferiority, or the stiff pelvis and weak legs, or the childhood trauma, or the sex-role attitudes, or whatever). What *is* important is that the whole cycle be dealt with, not just a single aspect of it. But how?

A 10-point "program" follows, designed to help you reduce your fears and anxieties—and increase your sexuality and your capacity for loving. Sound like magic? Not really. But before we begin, it will help for you to understand something quite simple about the human bodymind.

There are two opposing tendencies within each of us, which take different forms on different "levels" of existence. On the sexual level, they are anxiety and sexuality. On the muscular level, they are tension and relaxation. On the nervous system level, they are the sympathetic and parasympathetic subdivisions of the autonomic nervous system (these will be explained shortly). On the emotional level, and in the broadest sense as the two opposing forces within a personality, they are *fear* and *love.*

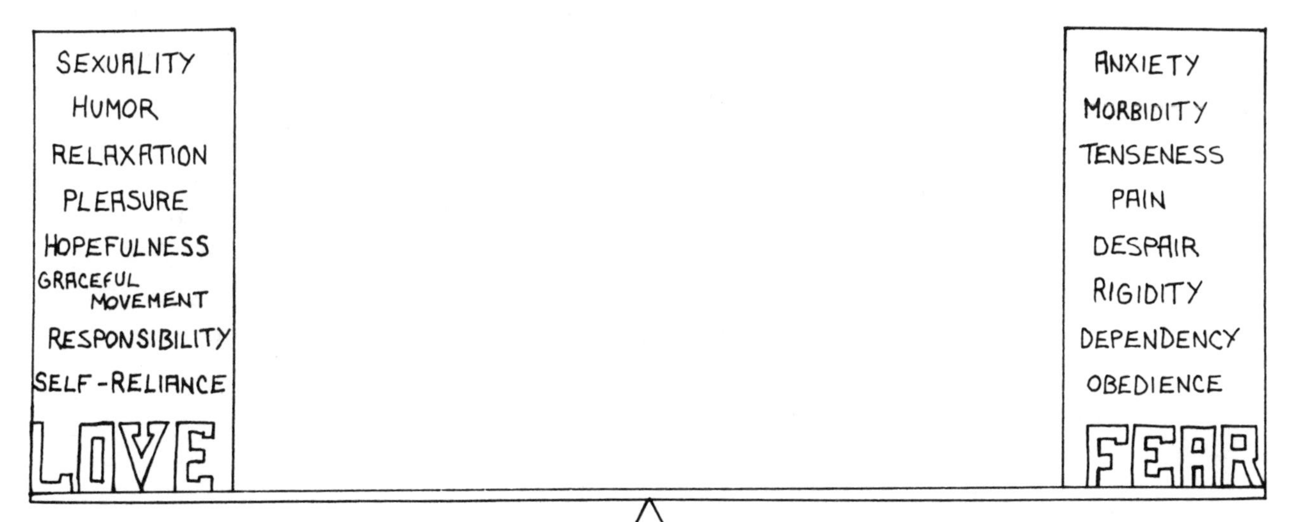

We can call fear the basic *negative* emotion; associated with it are the bodymind conditions of cruelty, hatred, anxiety, greed, despair, weakness, tension, dependency, and pain. And we can call love the basic *positive* emotion; its forms are affection, compassion, kindness, tolerance, hopefulness, generosity, responsibility, dynamic relaxation, fluid and graceful energy, openness, humor, sexuality, and pleasure. The positive and negative forces oppose each other continuously in every bodymind.

The autonomic nervous system controls all those organs, tissues, and processes that are involuntary—that is, the bodymind functions over which you generally have no control. The autonomic nervous system controls digestion, heartbeat and blood pressure, glandular secretions, sexual arousal, circulation of blood, healing processes, and so on. There are two subdivisions of this system, the sympathetic and the parasympathetic.

The sympathetic is essentially an emergency mechanism that prepares you for "fight or flight" when triggered by significant fear, pain, or threat. Its action constricts the blood vessels, raises heart rate and blood pressure, desensitizes the skin, stops the digestive processes, and also cuts off stimulation and circulation in the genital area. Sympathetic system functioning is associated with pain, anxiety, stress of all kinds—and the action of the will. It is a useful mechanism built into us by nature. In the event of combat or extreme danger, blood is withdrawn from the periphery of the body and concentrated for emergency use, nonessential functions are inhibited, and all energies are employed in overcoming or escaping the danger. Unfortunately, most of us walk, work, drive, and conduct our business in a state of at least partial sympathetic system action—in fact, whenever you do something that doesn't really *feel good,* the mechanism is on. (You're driving to work, for example, on a hot July day and you're stuck in slow traffic and feeling trapped and incredibly uncomfortable. What you'd most like to do is get off the highway, drive to a cool lake, dive in, and just glide through the luxuriantly cool water. But by an effort of the will, remembering your responsibilities and worried about what might happen if you actually *did* skip work that day, you repress your more natural feelings and keep on going. The result is that you wind up in what is actually a bodymind state of emergency—for most of your waking hours. The strain this puts on all aspects of your health, including your sexual response, is quite debilitating—but avoidable.)

The alternative to all this is the parasympathetic nervous system. The parasympathetic dilates the blood vessels, brings blood to the surface of the skin (increasing sensitivity), slows the heart rate, lowers blood pressure, controls digestion of food, and promotes sexual arousal and orgasm. Its operation is associated with feelings of pleasure, sexuality, confidence, and relaxation. Obviously, if you are anxious, fearful, or under some stress that has triggered the functioning of your sympathetic nervous system, this is going to make it much harder for you to feel pleasure, to relax, to be sexually responsive, and so on. (But surely you knew this before I told you?)

Our task, therefore, is to minimize the occasions when the sympathetic nervous system is operating, and maximize the functioning of the parasympathetic. Or, in more human terms, to reduce our fears and increase our loving. Here's how you might do it.

The 10-Point Program to Turn Fear into Love

Energy

You can't do anything without energy. I talked about Aerobic exercise and other forms of movement in Chapter One of this section. You have to do it, you have to feel the blood coursing through your body, feel the air rushing in and out of your lungs, feel your bodymind moving the way it was meant to move. You need energy for sex, and for loving. Tired, weary people are less attractive and less interesting than those with a living, vital energy. You can create a surplus of energy for yourself through plenty of natural movement and natural breathing. Why not do it?

Relaxation

Since we've already talked about relaxation, I just want to remind you of the importance of *letting go* whenever tensions and problems build up. Lie down or sit or walk and let yourself become calm, take a hot bath or do some Yoga or have someone you like give you a massage or do whatever it is that will relax you. Getting angry, when appropriate, is also relaxing; don't be afraid to express your anger! And, regularly every day, whether you are aware of your tensions and troubles or not, set aside a half hour for relaxation. This can be any time—before going to sleep, when you get home from work, even first thing in the morning. But do it every day—give yourself that half hour of solitude and peace and total self-concern. You could meditate during this time, or walk by a river, or just lie down and listen to some favorite piece of music. Let your worries subside for a while, and relax. It's good for you.

Awareness

Try to become aware of those factors that block your energy and make you tense and anxious. Start from a good place—after a long run, or a beautiful sexual experience, or an hour of Yoga and a hot shower. Start from a point where you feel "right"—relaxed, happy, centered, unhassled, and healthy. And then observe yourself. Keep track and try to find out *at what moment* you start to lose that relaxed-energetic feeling. When do your shoulder muscles start to tighten up? When do your buttocks become deadened again? When do your spirits fall? Keep track of yourself, and when you start to lose it—whether that occasion is a remark by someone else, an unfamiliar social situation, a memory or an idea or a worry, or some physical event like a sudden change in temperature or stubbing your toe—*stop.* Don't let yourself be made uptight or unhappy by such minor circumstances! Recall the relaxed and happy state of bodymind you were in just a little while ago, remember the feeling and get it back. It's not so hard because you were just there. Now try to maintain your state of health right through whatever difficulty or stress you are encountering. You can do it. And whenever you find yourself feeling uptight, anxious, frightened, or otherwise imbalanced or in pain, remember your "right" bodymind pattern and get back to it. Sometimes this will only require taking a few deep breaths; sometimes it will mean consciously letting go of your shoulders, so that the tension goes out of them; or you may want to shut your eyes for a few seconds. Sometimes it will mean getting mad for a little while, and letting out some righteous anger. But if you can possibly avoid it, don't allow yourself to be "put off" by circumstances, whatever they are—because you have within you a state of positive, relaxed, confident, and energetic health.

Become *aware* of how your system works, and what kinds of things cause fear and tension and pain to set in. Then you can prevent them, and maintain that state of health and energy always.

Honesty

Go on an honesty kick with yourself. What are you feeling? What do you want? What is obstructing you from being happy, or fulfilled, or loving? What needs and desires of yours are not being met—and why? Most people who are dissatisfied or unhealthy are that way because they are out of touch with themselves. They don't even admit to themselves, much less give expression to, their real needs and desires. This is why those needs are never met, why people become sick emotionally and physically. Wilhelm Reich held that there are several *primary drives* in the human organism—such as movement, sexuality, and love—and that when these basic drives are frustrated, repressed, or denied, they produce the negative *secondary drives*—hatred, sadism, dependency, violence, and so on. If you examine your own behavior carefully, you'll see how true this is. The first step is to *admit* your needs; then you might actually find them getting met.

Nonthinking

You think too much! You don't sense enough, feel enough, move enough, or breathe enough. You get so accustomed to having your mind run the show that you can't turn it off and operate on another basis, even when you want to. This is especially true of people with "sex problems." They can't devote themselves totally to the physical-emotional here and now of making love. Instead, they are thinking of one thing or another—a person other than the one they are with, an appointment they forgot to keep, whether they left the door unlocked, anxiety about their "performance." And because of this thinking they are unable to be really "there," to enjoy the moment and respond fully to another person. Good sex is premised upon utter abandonment to primitive, unconscious, natural forces and feelings. The conscious, "thinking" mind can only interfere with this most basic process, and diminish its intensity, if not destroy it. Probably you realize this already. But what is to be done when your mind *does* interfere, when you are thinking overtime and can't enjoy yourself, sexually or otherwise, because you are burdened by all your "other" fears, insecurities, and troubles?

Practice nonthinking. There are many ways to do this. Meditation is a good one. Really getting into music is another—especially making your own music. Dancing is good nonthinking, especially if you just move to the music and forget everything else. Any kind of really strenuous activity—like hiking up a mountain—will make you do less thinking and more feeling, more *being*. Working with your hands—on clay, on wood, on bodies —reduces your mind's dominance. Feel around for your own ways. By getting reaccustomed to nonthinking modes of experience, you will then find it easier to give yourself up to the feelings of love, and lovemaking. Do it—don't think about it!

List your fears

Fear and love are like the two ends of a seesaw—as one goes down, the other goes up. It's hard to feel affectionate and sexy and centered and generous when you're frightened or in pain or worried. On the other hand, when you're in a relaxed, energetic, sexually fulfilled and loving state, you're much less likely to react with fear, panic, anxiety, or repressed anger to whatever difficulties befall you. Fear is the crippler, the obstructor, the real cause of almost every disease, every injustice, every disorder of body and mind.

All too often we are witness to the terrible violence and cruelty that human beings inflict upon one another —not out of any innate evil or "killer instinct"—but as externalizations of their own fear and pain. We don't have to look at history, at the war-racked world and the countless social and political horrors of our time, to verify this. Just look at yourself, and at those you know well. When do you act selfishly, cruelly, inconsiderately? When do things "go wrong" for you, instead of going right? When do you hate? When do you get sick, when do you feel weak, when do you destroy or want to destroy? When do you fail to enjoy life in its simplest forms—so that you eat but are not nourished, you sleep but are not rested, you go through the act of love but are not fulfilled?

When do these things happen? When you are *afraid.* What kinds of things are people afraid of? Physical pain, obviously. Losing someone you love—or losing someone's love. Losing property, or other wealth that you have worked hard to gain. Being humiliated, disgraced, rejected, ridiculed. Being defeated at anything. Giving up an image of yourself. Not succeeding in your chosen work. Becoming old or becoming ill, and being a burden on others. Dying. People fear so many things. What are *you* afraid of?

The first and most important step in overcoming your fears is simply to admit them. You will see that many fears are trivial or unwarranted, not worth your distress. And the others, the two or three or half-dozen major fears you have that cannot be dismissed so easily—these especially should be admitted, examined, put into a simple form so that you can face them without panic or weakness. Do it now. Be honest! Take a sheet of paper and write down everything you are afraid of.

Be sure to list everything, from the most insignificant, minor worry to the most impossible and terrifying fear of your life. No one else need ever see this list. But you should see it. It will be a relief just to look at your fears; and it may be a new beginning. Take five minutes now and do this. You can never eliminate your fears until you bring them out into the open and acknowledge them.

Do something you're afraid of ________________________

Karate and the other Oriental martial arts (Kung Fu, Aikido, Jujutsu, T'ai Chi Ch'uan, etc.) are really, in essence, systems of alchemy from negative to positive—that is, from cruelty, unnatural anger, greed, weakness, fear, and despair, to compassion, relaxation, openness, confidence, love, and power. A great deal of time and energy is devoted to fear—in fact, the entire art of Karate (or T'ai Chi or any of the others) might be considered the elimination of fear from the whole bodymind.

We start with smaller fears—such as the fear of fighting to defend yourself, the fear of falling, the fear of getting hit or of hitting something. After a while, in the course of training, deeper fears are confronted—the fear of being a coward, fear of facing oneself honestly and without illusion, fear of giving up old habits of the bodymind for the sake of something new, fear of losing—ultimately, even the fear of dying. For almost all of these the mechanism used to eliminate them is to *go through the fear,* that is, do the very thing you are afraid of: to break a board, to fight with someone much bigger and stronger than you, to take a punch in the jaw—and see that it's not nearly so bad as the fear itself.

This is no easy task. It explains why so few people really pursue the martial arts into their deeper levels, although many take them up, and learn how to make a few kicks or throw a few punches. But the most difficult aspect is always facing yourself and working through your fears. I recommend it for everyone, whether you're a martial artist or not. There's no greater feeling than to actually do something you were afraid of—and, regardless of whether you "win" or "lose," to eliminate that fear forever from your life.

The great Positive Energy has many names, *ki, ch'i, prana,* orgone, life-force—these are just a few of them. There are also many ways to bring it out in your own life, and into the world. Breathing practice is a way—filling yourself with prana from the air you breathe. Centering practice is another way, because the ch'i spreads through your whole bodymind from Hara. All forms of relaxation, which means the removing of obstacles, can release the flow of life within you. (Remember that tension is fear-in-your-body.) Getting close to nature is good. Look for the life in all things, and don't be afraid. *Feel* life in yourself, at all times; this is the most important thing. Nothing is worth your fear, not even death. But a great many things are worth your work, your energy, your commitment, your struggle —and your love.

If fear is the trap and the prison of this life, then love is the way out. Love is the order of the universe as it flows within us, and it is the force that heals. Lose everything, and you may still have love; let the world crumble, yet love remains. Because love is movement, love is breath. Love is supple, yielding yet remaining whole. Love is in all things that live—the ant, the grass, the fish, the tree. Love is the seed, the womb, the joining, the planting. It is the baby, the child, the man, the woman.

The ways of love are many. Anything you do well, that feels good and benefits the world, is a way. Music is good, dancing, singing, poetry, walking, making things, running, embracing, laughing—all the human arts are love. Close your eyes and feel your own life. That's it. Keep the juice turned on. There's all you need. Life is in you.

Relate to someone else

You don't want to live alone. You want to be known—and to know others. All those fears and all those desires you have now admitted to yourself and are doing something about—how much better if you can tell them to someone. How much better if you can work them through by becoming involved with a bodymind other than your own. Any honest attempt to live with and understand another person is a way of growth and an unfolding of life-energy, at least as much as any system you might undertake. A real, open, honest, joyful giving-and-receiving sexual relationship is one of the most beautiful and human of ways. But how could I presume to tell you exactly how you should go about such a thing? It's a great and awesome mystery to me! But I do know it's real.

Clothing and nakedness

This last one is easy: Go naked as much as you can, and wear loose, comfortable clothes the rest of the time. Ties and tight shoes and belts and corsets and tight pants and all the other things people wear for fashion's sake, or just out of habit—these can cut down your circulation, cut off feeling to certain parts of you, divide you up unnaturally, restrict and inhibit your free movement, alter your normal posture, not to mention making you just plain uncomfortable.

Unfortunately our society is still so backward as to lock people up for appearing nude in public (even in hot weather!), so you'll have to keep your nakedness out of the public eye. This does not mean out of the open air, however. Even going around naked at home is good for you; it lets the so-called private parts breathe. And, really, dress yourself for your own comfort and health and relaxation first—and for society's sake second. Okay?

Don't get me wrong. I don't mean to be giving you instructions on how to live. I myself am a student of life, a traveler, a warrior, a householder just like you. But I hate to see so many people missing out on all the sexual enjoyment and loving health that is theirs if they just let it out. That's really why I wrote this book.

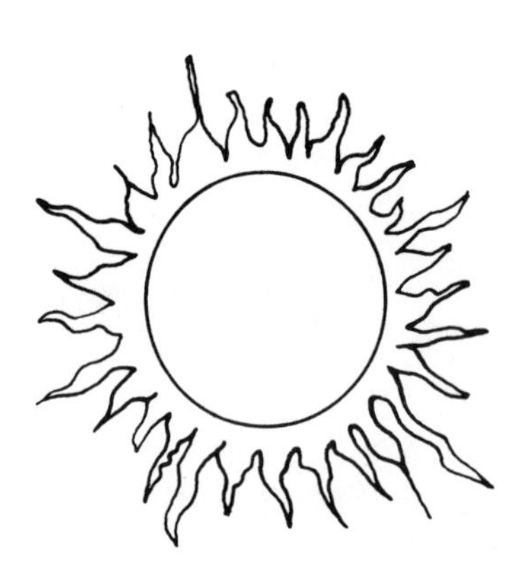

FOOD

> What a strange machine man is! You fill him with bread, wine, fish, radishes, and out of him come sighs, laughter, and dreams.
>
> KAZANTZAKIS, *Zorba the Greek*

A strange and mysterious machine, all right! Some people eat only brown rice, you know, and thrive. Some folks eat only meat, and are strong. Some eat only fruit and leafy vegetables. Some eat hot dogs and candy bars. All manage to survive.

The doctors, the dietitians, the nutritionists, the fanatical advocates of one set of dietary rules and principles or another—most of them don't live any longer, run any faster, or seem any happier or any healthier than a lot of ordinary people who just live well and don't think about food too much. Mind you, I'm not saying that a sugary candy bar is just as good for you as a piece of fresh, ripe fruit—of course it isn't. Nor am I saying that there are not such things as general human needs for certain vitamins, minerals, and other nutrients essential to healthy physical-and-mental functioning —certainly there are.

But what you eat means a great deal. It's rarely just what happens to be available at a particular time, or what you happen to feel like consuming. Your food patterns, like your posture, your breathing, and all your physical characteristics, reflect both the long-term and short-term patterns in your personality, and your life-style. Tackling the food question is really no less than tackling the whole life question; it's just another way to go about it.

For example: In our culture most children are brought up to associate sweet, sugary foods (candy, cake, gum, soda) as synonymous with affection, goodness, and love. This is the inevitable result of a simple conditioning process: The child does something "good" and he is rewarded with a sweet; or he's told to "do this for me and I'll buy you a chocolate bar"; or at his birthday party the main attraction is—the cake; and so it goes.

This conditioning becomes an internal pattern in the person, lasting into adulthood. Thus when the grown-up person feels lonely, or bored, or in need of reinforcement, he (or she) goes to the refrigerator for a piece of cake, or puts a dime in the nearest candy machine. By this time the whole thing has become a sort of physical *addiction:* The sugar in the sweet stuff *does* give a temporary raising of energy, which *feels* good—thus reinforcing the need for sweet and rooting the whole association in the body itself. Needless to say, white sugar and all the products made with it are no good for you. Refined sugar and refined sugar products can produce tooth decay, gum diseases, obesity, hypoglycemia (low blood sugar), diabetes—and contribute to vitamin B deficiency and other nutritional imbalances.

What happens is that a very unnatural conditioned association replaces your natural instinct for right food. Naturally, you seek quick energy from the other forms of sugar—glucose, fructose, lactose, maltose—found in such natural foods as (respectively) honey, fresh fruits, milk, germinated grains. The cultural conditioning substitutes unhealthy refined (white *or* brown) sugar for this normal hunger for energy-giving substances.

Breaking the wrong-food pattern involves breaking

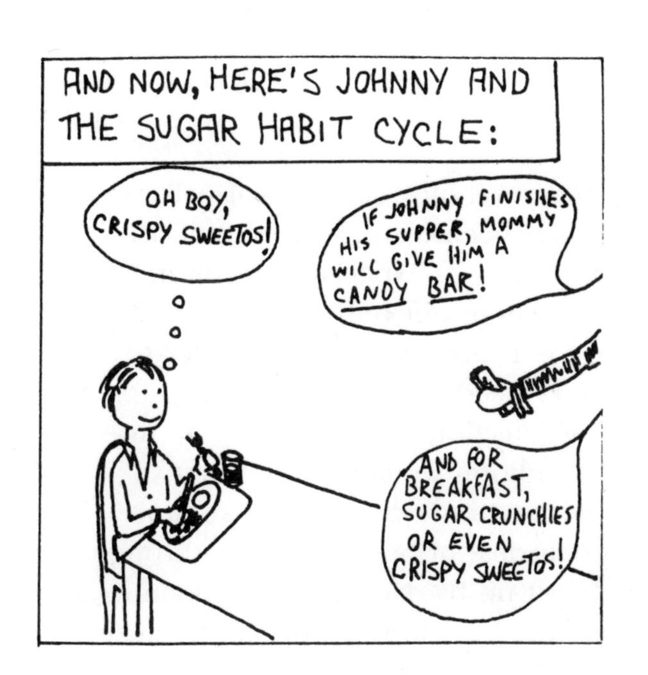
AND NOW, HERE'S JOHNNY AND THE SUGAR HABIT CYCLE:
OH BOY, CRISPY SWEETOS!
IF JOHNNY FINISHES HIS SUPPER, MOMMY WILL GIVE HIM A CANDY BAR!
AND FOR BREAKFAST, SUGAR CRUNCHIES OR EVEN CRISPY SWEETOS!

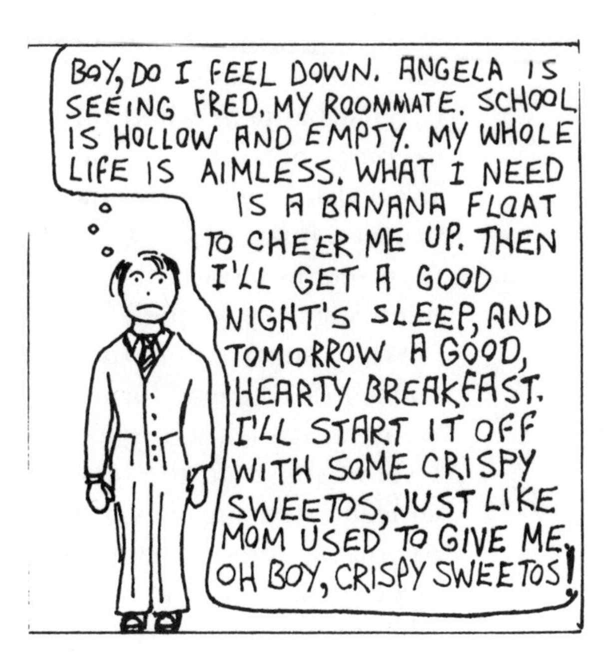
BOY, DO I FEEL DOWN. ANGELA IS SEEING FRED, MY ROOMMATE. SCHOOL IS HOLLOW AND EMPTY. MY WHOLE LIFE IS AIMLESS. WHAT I NEED IS A BANANA FLOAT TO CHEER ME UP. THEN I'LL GET A GOOD NIGHT'S SLEEP, AND TOMORROW A GOOD, HEARTY BREAKFAST. I'LL START IT OFF WITH SOME CRISPY SWEETOS, JUST LIKE MOM USED TO GIVE ME. OH BOY, CRISPY SWEETOS!

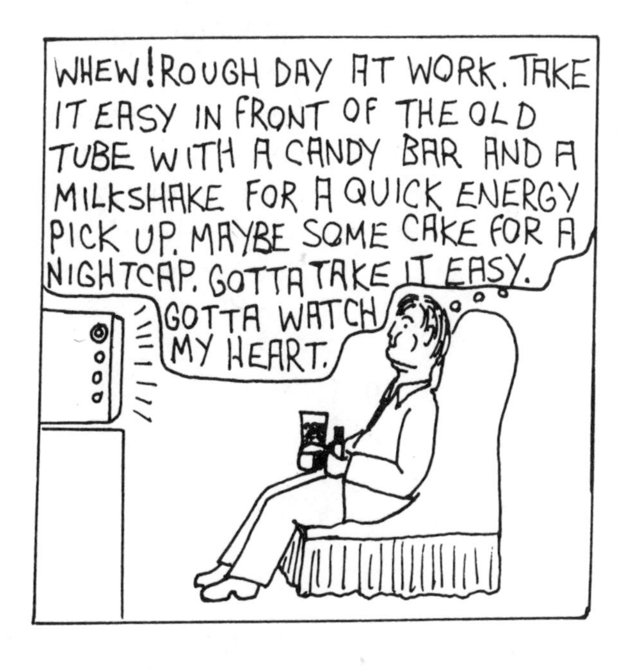
WHEW! ROUGH DAY AT WORK. TAKE IT EASY IN FRONT OF THE OLD TUBE WITH A CANDY BAR AND A MILKSHAKE FOR A QUICK ENERGY PICK UP. MAYBE SOME CAKE FOR A NIGHTCAP. GOTTA TAKE IT EASY. GOTTA WATCH MY HEART.

that whole deep-rooted psychological-physical pattern of emotional needs that has been turned into the desire for sweet foods. This pattern is especially strong in overweight people, for whom not only sweets but all kinds of high-caloric foods are consumed in order to satisfy other, nondietary needs.

An example of food selection determined by an immediate, short-term condition would be the thirst of a man who has been working outside on a hot summer day. Having lost a great deal of body moisture through perspiration, he makes it up by drinking great quantities of liquids. This is natural and entirely normal, because we have a thirst instinct: When the body's moisture level drops, we feel the desire for water. But for pure water only—that's what thirst is about.

What happens when this natural thirst for water becomes perverted by the cultural conditioning for sweet drinks, like carbonated soda pop? The thirsty man drinks a quart of Coke or Pepsi or Seven Up—which then sets in motion the whole *refined sugar cycle.* The refined sugar cycle goes like this:

White sugar enters the bloodstream as sucrose, a very concentrated sugar form not found in nature. The pancreas, which is the organ in your body that regulates the level of sugars in the blood, responds to this highly concentrated sugar as if it were a dangerous overdose to your system—it panics, overreacts, and produces large quantities of insulin to counteract this overdose. The insulin neutralizes not only the refined sugar you have just consumed but also some of your other essential blood sugars. This leaves you with a *low* blood sugar condition! Low blood sugar means more fatigue and less energy than before you consumed the sugary product. If this cycle is set in motion when you least need it—as in the example of the thirsty man in the middle of a hard day's work—and your energy level goes way down, you may be in trouble.

Another example of natural needs versus cultural conditioning: You sit down for lunch, nervous and anxious because a really difficult job awaits you at work later in the afternoon. Your nervousness has made your stomach nervous too, and you're not really sure you want to eat anything at all. This is quite a normal reaction—stress, anxiety, nervous anticipation all naturally inhibit the appetite. It's a very primitive thing—as an animal, if you have to fight or take flight, you do better to be light and quick, not weighted down by heavy food. (The flow of blood to your stomach for digestion leaves less blood for your muscles to move with, and less for your brain to think with; it makes you slow and dull.) So what do you do? Most people, unfortunately, don't listen to the messages of their own bodies. They just go ahead and eat anyway. They don't enjoy the meal, they don't benefit from it, probably they get indigestion—at the very least they feel much less on top of things than before they ate. Having that lunch "anyway" only makes you less able to deal with the problem; and may produce even more anxiety, nervousness, and physical upset. *Missing* the meal, on the other hand, wouldn't hurt you in the least!

The problem goes further than this. Every feeling, every action, every thought is also a chemical and electrical event inside your body. This is why taking a certain drug can make you feel different, putting you in a relaxed mood, or making you hyperactive and energetic, or even altering your thinking processes in some way. It's why the brain waves of Zen monks during deep meditation are slower and more regular (the Alpha wave pattern) than the brain waves of normally conscious, busy, slightly nervous people (Beta wave pattern). It's why sometimes you have a great desire for acid foods (vinegar, apples, citrus) if you've been very active—because your body's chemical balance becomes more acid (less alkaline) during exertion. Sometimes you crave foods rich in vitamin C (orange juice, berries, tomatoes), especially after periods of stress or after drinking or smoking a lot—stress and toxic substances deplete your body's store of C, which has to be replenished. Sometimes you may crave dairy products such as milk, cheese, or yoghurt, reflecting your body's need for more calcium.

The point is that your system is in a continuous state of change: using up various elements for various purposes; transporting foodstuffs to certain parts of the body; carrying waste products away; breaking down certain compounds, synthesizing others from internally-available materials; secreting tiny amounts of powerful substances into the bloodstream that have been produced by the ductless glands; getting rid of unusable substances through sweat, urine, and feces; rushing blood to different organs or muscles for movement, thought, digestion, emotional response, sexual activity, sensitivity, and so on.

Some foods meet the needs demanded by these changes—and some do not. Some foods meet immediate needs, like water to relieve dehydration. Some foods meet long-term needs, like high-protein foods (meat, fish, cheese, etc.) used for building new cells, repairing damaged tissue, and as reserve source of energy. And some foods may actually be harmful to you and work contrary to the needs of your body—even be poisonous in one degree or another.

No diet is appropriate to all people at all times and under all circumstances! The variables are too immense. Each person's chemistry is different, their characters are different, their ways of living are different—and their diets must also be different. But if there is no fixed dietary principle that will be good for everyone, how do you go about determining what you should eat?

First, a few common-sense suggestions:

1. Try to avoid refined sugar and all foods made with it—candies, cakes, sodas, and a thousand other products (read the labels!). This includes brown sugar as well as white—sorry, all you brown-sugar lovers. Brown sugar is only white sugar with some of the molasses put back in! One hundred years ago our healthy ancestors in this country consumed about 5 pounds of sugar per person per year. Today the average American adult consumes close to *150 pounds* of sugar per year! (Put that in your coffee and stir it.)
2. Try to avoid highly refined and processed foods such as white-flour products, most breakfast cereals, TV dinners, white rice, frozen desserts, and other things like that (again, read them labels!).

   Despite their advertising claims of "added vitamins," most of these refined and processed foods are nutritionally deficient—they lack the most essential parts and are loaded with harmful chemicals (preservatives, bleaching agents, softeners, artificial flavoring and coloring, and lots more). Regular white flour, for example, has had the bran and the germ removed, which are the two most valuable parts of the wheat! (The bran and germ are then sold to drug companies, which sell them back to you as vitamin and mineral supplements —at tremendous prices!) Try instead to eat whole-grain cereals (brown rice, whole wheat bread, whole oats), freshly cooked meats and vegetables, raw fruits, and other natural products. If something has to be cooked, you do much better to cook it yourself, starting from the raw stuff as Nature produced it!
3. Try to get fruits and vegetables that have not been sprayed with pesticides, insecticides, and fungicides; that have not been grown with chemical fertilizers, from chemically-treated seeds; that have not been covered with wax, or paraffin, or artificial coloring. Get "*organic*" fruits and vegetables! They're richer in vitamins and minerals than regular commercial foods. They won't slowly poison you with DDT, parathion, dieldrin, and a thousand other toxic chemical additives. And they actually taste better.
4. Cut down on coffee, tea (except herb teas, which have no tannic acid), cigarettes, sweet drinks, pills, pot, alcohol—any-

thing you may take into your system regularly that in the long run won't do you any good. If you're tired, for example, you should rest—not drink a cup of coffee to keep you going. On the other hand, your tiredness might be mental, might be from *lack* of physical activity, in which case a brisk walk is in order—not a pep pill. *Try the natural way.* It may take a little getting used to at first, but it pays off.

5. Unless you've already attained such a high level of personal development that nothing in this world ever bothers you, you never get upset, you have no problems, and are never under any stress of any kind (if you *are* such a person, drop me a line!)—you probably need some amount of vitamin C over and above that of your everyday diet. Stress, anxiety, the poisons in the air, water, and food—all of these use up your body's store of C. It seems that there's more stress and more deadly substances being consumed by man today than he is equipped by nature to handle, especially on a refined and unnatural diet. So it may be very likely that you need some vitamin C supplements. You should determine this *for yourself,* by trial and error. Take some every day for a month, say, and see if you notice any improvement in your general condition. You can determine the dosage in the same way—don't worry, it's next to impossible to overdose on C.
6. *Don't eat when you're not hungry.* Your body is sending you a message, which you should heed! Don't eat a big meal if you have a lot of work (physical or mental) to do afterwards—digesting food concentrates a lot of blood in the stomach and intestines, leaving much less available for the brain and the musculature.

   Meat-eating animals (carnivores) like the lion, the python, the bear, usually eat a huge amount and are immobilized for at least several hours while digesting it. Plant-eating animals (herbivores) such as the deer, the horse, and the giraffe eat almost continually of small quantities of relatively light food—they browse, that is. The carnivorous eating pattern is feasible only if you can afford to sleep off that big meal—or at least relax for an hour with a good magazine. The herbivorous eating pattern may be more suitable than two or three huge meals, especially if you've got a full day's work to do. The best thing is to find your own best eating pattern, whatever it is.
7. Drink some clear, pure water every day—preferably three or four glasses, or more. Water is essential to your system for cleansing, for elimination, for the quality of the blood, and for maintaining the right internal chemical balance in all your

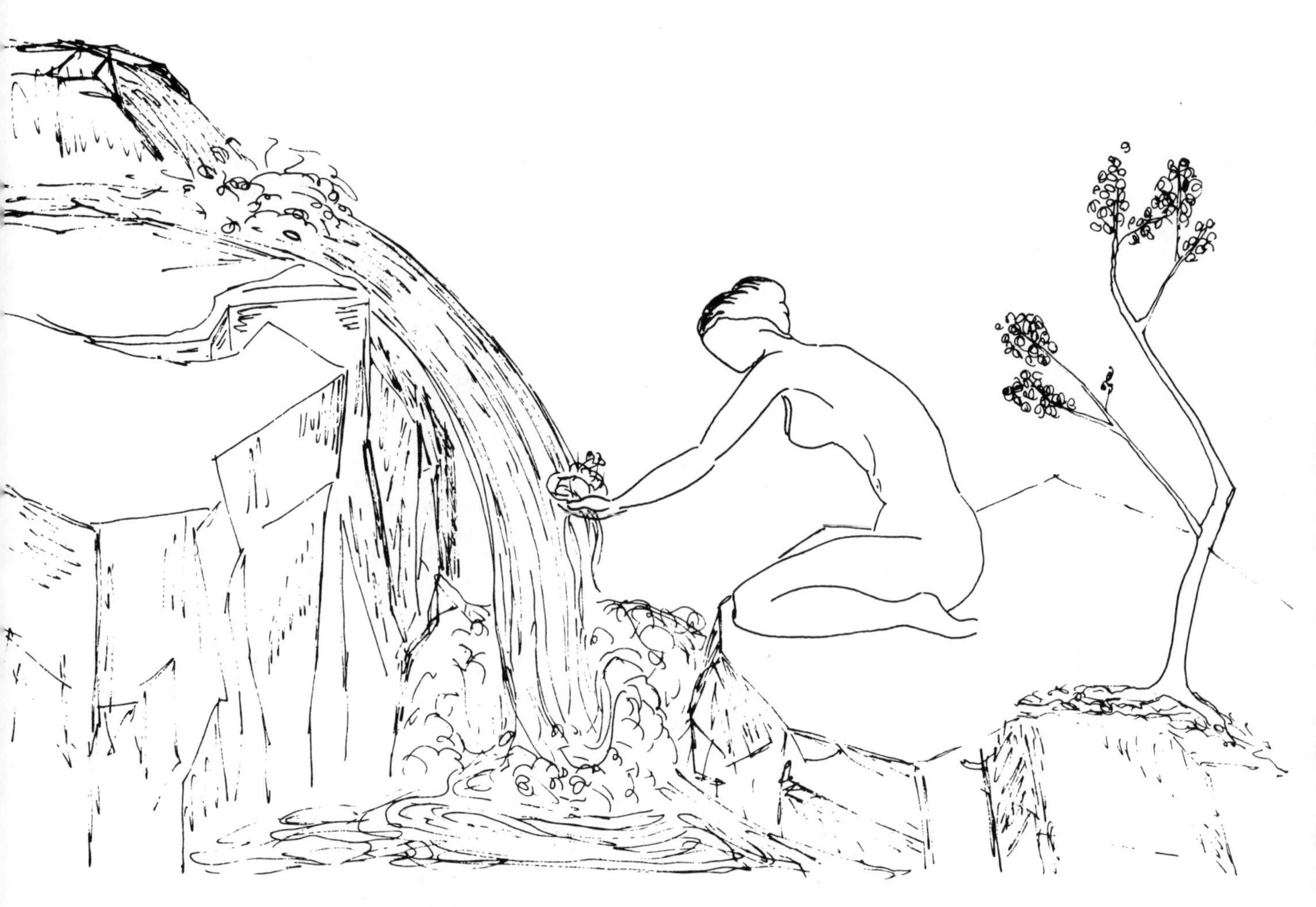

organs. There is nothing that can replace it. (Especially if you have stomach or intestinal troubles!) If you sweat a great deal, or whenever you feel thirsty—*drink water.* If your tap water is not pure, either boil it or get fresh spring water or well water. There's no better drink in the world than sweet, fresh water!

So much for common sense. In Part III, I outline several of the major dietary systems (Macrobiotic, Mucusless, Natural-Organic, etc.) and discuss their theories, methods, and prescriptions. In addition to these, there are a thousand and one reducing diets, athletic training diets, Yoga diets, high-protein diets, low-car-

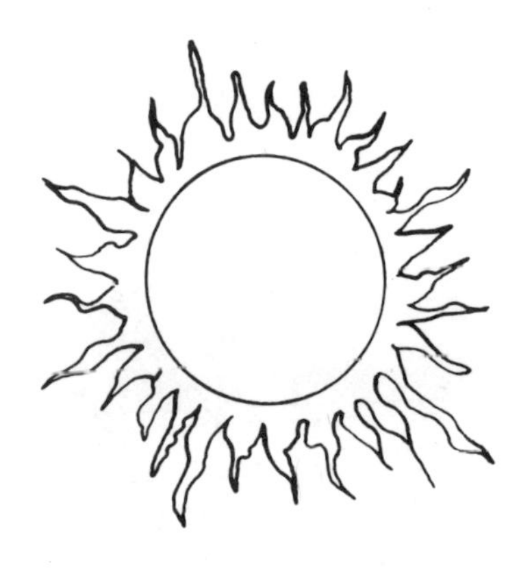

bohydrate diets, mono diets, low-salt diets, raw foods diets—all with their own virtues and their own flaws. Some people spend their lives going from one of these diets to the next, always hoping for the perfect one that will make them healthier. That's not the way to do it! What we need now is a way to determine our own special needs with respect to food. Are you with me?

Every living creature is equipped by nature with a *food instinct*—a built-in, unconscious mechanism that tells the animal what things are food and what things are not food. The food instinct may also make the animal aware of what particular type of food to eat at any particular time, as its needs change. The human animal is also equipped with a food instinct—only it is distorted, buried, deflected, even destroyed by our culture, with its strange faith in thinking as *the* solution to all of our problems—and its rejection, suppression, and mistrust of all that is instinctual, sensual, and animal in human nature.

Here's the proof: Infants (up to the age of perhaps one or two years, depending on their upbringing) given a free choice between healthy, natural foods and artificial, processed foods, will invariably pick the food that is best for them! Without fail, babies pick fresh fruit, lean meat (especially organ meats such as liver), and raw vegetables over white bread, candy, pastries, ice cream, overcooked vegetables.

Several years later, though, when the societal conditioning has begun to set in and the natural instincts have already been buried, they'll choose the artificial foods over the natural ones. (What six-year-old do you know who will pick a piece of raw liver over a Mars bar?) And most adults, as well, repeat this unhealthy choice of the artificial over the natural in their daily lives—disregarding the innate food instincts of their own bodies. *True health in relation to food is not the diligent following of any particular diet, but the rediscovery of your own food instinct.*

How do you go about doing this?

First, by improving your overall health in the ways I've already described—plenty of natural movement, deep breathing, flexibility, relaxation, the reestablishment of the Hara (lower center), and emotional and sexual fulfillment. All these things serve to rekindle the instinctual mechanisms within you.

Second, by breaking your habitual, conditioned eating patterns with a brief fast. (See the instructions in Part III on how to begin fasting.) Fasting will improve your general condition in a number of ways—it helps eliminate many toxic substances from your body; it rests and rejuvenates your digestive system; and it clears your mind of many of its habits and prejudices with regard to food. Most importantly, fasting will bring your food instincts to the fore.

In the first day of a fast you may be drooling over the thought of hot-fudge sundaes and McDonald's superburgers and monstrous birthday cakes; this will pass. After not too long you'll look at a single apple and imagine you could live on it for a week, because there's so much *life* in it. What happens over a fast of some duration—three days at least—is that your *appetite* begins to disappear. Your appetite is your cultural-social-mental-emotional-taste bud desire for food, which appears at mealtimes and at certain other times—whether your body really requires any food or not, and whether the food you're going to eat is any good for you or not.

When your appetite fades, in its place returns *hunger.* Hunger is the basic, primitive, animal instinct to find and consume food—because your body needs it, and for no other reason! Most of us have not felt real hunger for a long time, if ever. But the healthy animal (human or any other kind) eats only at the demand of hunger—*not* to satisfy the appetite.

Return to the feeling of hunger by fasting, exercising, getting close to nature. Become really *aware* of what is food and what isn't. Keeping up a fast is not as hard as you might think; the first couple of meals you skip are by far the worst! And fasting is worth the effort. After a week (if you can make it that long), you won't need anyone to tell you what to eat! And when you do start eating again—even if your fast only lasted 24 hours—you'll know the feeling of eating food when you *need* it. Remember that feeling—anything else is unnatural appetite, not hunger, and it's probably not good for you.

You conscious mind can serve your food instincts in at least one helpful capacity: by identifying sprayed foods and chemically-treated products, distinguishing them from natural foods. Sometimes your instincts alone can't do this. A sprayed apple may look as attractive as an organically-grown one.

As your innate food instincts return, you will actually become able to tell commercially-grown, sprayed, and treated foods from natural, organically-grown ones—almost as easily as you can tell the difference between meat from domestic livestock and meat of wild game animals. Still, there are lots of tasteless, odorless, colorless additives that can escape even the the most rejuvenated of senses. Your brain comes in here, and directs you to the more wholesome stuff. Brains do have their uses!

In dealing with what you eat, the same pattern emerges as with all the other life functions we've been talking about:

1. You realize that the present situation is unsatisfactory and in need of improvement.
2. You consciously examine the problem and take certain steps to deal with it by consciously changing your ways. (In this case, let's say, you decide to eliminate highly refined and processed foods, cut out white sugar altogether, and try a three-day fast.)
3. Finally, you reach the point where you don't have to *think* about the function (whether it's breathing, eating, running, seeing, loving, or whatever) because your system instinctively does the right thing.

Good health is within you—it needs only to be freed. Regain your innate instinct and feeling for nourishing, natural food and you need never concern yourself with diet again!

One last note. Your body, as Zorba says, is a strange and wonderful machine. It is capable of taking an incredible variety of different substances and turning them into energy and flesh, expelling the unusable portions. The multitude of differing diets that humans live on around the world is proof of this fantastic capacity of the body. Eskimos eat blubber, Indians make flour from acorns, other people eat ants, flowers, shark fins, grasses—not to mention fungi (mushrooms!) and fish eggs (caviar!). With so many possible diets that can keep you alive, it's important to be relaxed, flexible, and noncompulsive about food—besides being natural and instinctual.

If someone cooks a meal for you with love, with care, with the beauty of their concern, eat it and enjoy it and be well nourished by it, whatever it is! In the final analysis it's these things—attitude, concern, environment, company, and emotion—that really determine the quality and the effect of food, not chemical formulas. So move, breathe, laugh, love, get hungry—and eat well!

MIND

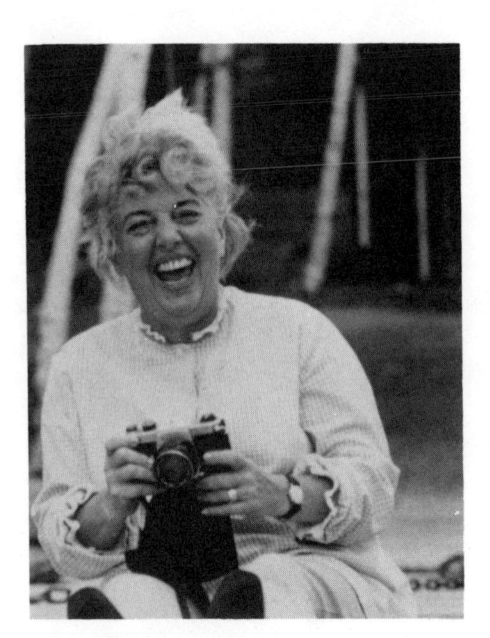

The author's mother in a contemplative mood

Is your mind the same thing as your brain? I don't think it is, exactly. The brain is gray matter (nerve tissue) charged with electrical energy in certain patterns that correspond to patterns of thought and behavior. But does this really explain the commonest train of thought, or dream, or flight of the imagination? Does it explain the great artistic, musical, and literary works of man? Can it account for ESP, clairvoyance, prophecy, and psychic phenomena of all kinds? Is some pattern of electrical impulses through a few pounds of gray matter the essential nature of the world-renewing spiritual experiences of such men as Jesus, Buddha, Mohammed, Lao Tzu?

What is the mind then? Most of the time we accept the definition of mind that is implied in the "mind-body" duality. That is, the "mind" is everything we can experience that is not purely physical. But, as I've been showing you all along, there is nothing that you can experience that is purely of the body, or purely of the mind. Instead, there's a constant interconnection and interrelationship between mind and body, which are more like the North and South poles of the same globe than two separate and exclusive realms. The healthier you become, the more "together" your mind and body get to be—until finally they form a single, united entity: the bodymind of the whole person.

Let me illustrate this with an example from the martial arts. In Karate there is a blocking technique known as Rising Block (used to ward off a strike to the head), and a punching technique called Reverse Punch (which employs the full twisting movement of the hips to generate tremendous force). Together the two techniques form a simple and effective defense and counterattack to any straight or downward blow to the head, either with fist, club, knife, stick, or any other weapon.

The beginning Karate student first learns how to execute the techniques properly on his own—that is, as movements practiced in the air, not as responses to any threatened attack by another person. Like shadowboxing, there is no opponent, only the technique to be learned and improved. It may take months, even years, before the block and punch are flawless—quick, precise, and powerful. The student's body must acquire a form of moving that it did not have before; this demands long, endlessly repetitious practice.

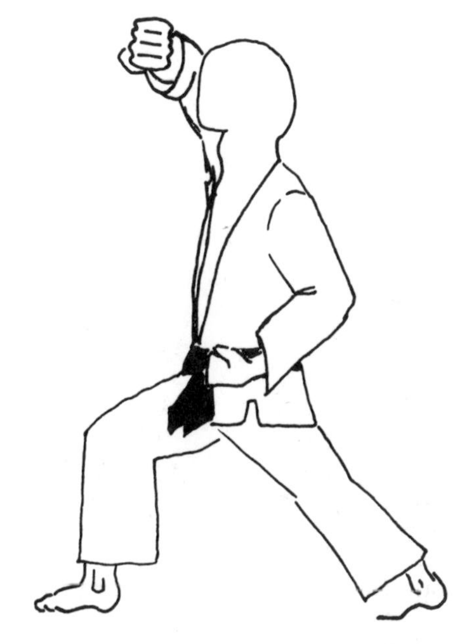

Rising Block

Some time later, the block and punch are practiced as a defense against a realistic attack made by another Karate student in a prearranged situation. The "attacker" indicates he is going to take a step and punch to the "defender's" head. The defender decides beforehand that he is going to practice the Rising Block and Reverse Punch in response to this assault. In this case a limited element of actual danger is introduced—if the defender fails to block the attack he *may* be hit in the face. Nevertheless, the usefulness of the block-and-punch technique *as a necessity* becomes apparent. The student may temporarily falter at this point in performing the movements he has learned to do so well when practicing on his own; but again, with perseverance, he gains the use of his techniques in the simulated attack situation.

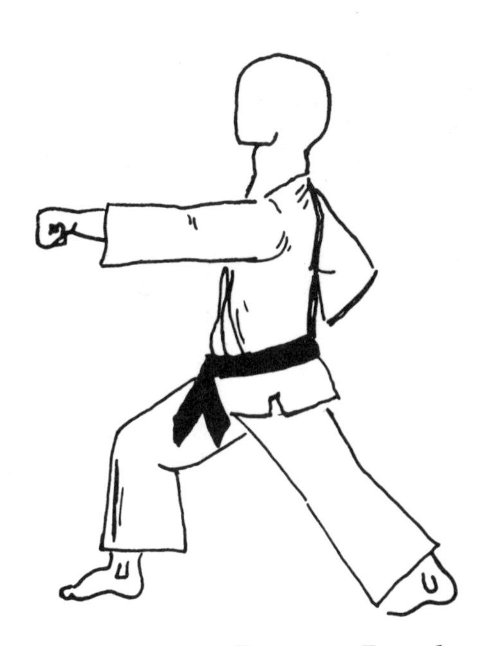

Reverse Punch

At a later stage in his training, the student is called upon to use this particular block-punch combination, when appropriate, in the even more realistic practice of free-style sparring with another student. In this case nothing is prearranged, and the movements and responses must be spontaneous, swift, and decisive. Punches, kicks, and strikes are freely exchanged (although stopped just short of their target or else landed without force) and must be met with appropriate blocking, shifting, and counterattacking responses. If the student uses his basic block-and-punch technique here, it must be executed with great speed and perfect accuracy, for both the threat and the target are a moving, thinking, seeing person.

The actual use of the Rising Block-Reverse Punch combination in a life-and-death situation may never occur. The training, the practice, the perseverance, the self-discipline, and the concentration necessary to master the technique have been themselves reward enough for the serious martial artist. And if the Karate man has trained properly, there will never be a problem in applying what he has learned: When the necessity truly arises, then the right technique "happens"—instantaneously, reflexively, without a moment's hesitation or thought. Perceiving a dangerous attack, selecting the appropriate response, and executing the defense and counterattack all occur in the same split second. At the level of true mastery, we may say that these three elements are the same single event. This is the higher level of bodymind unity.

Can we really say that there has been a separation of mind and body during this training process? All along, the student's task has not been just to acquire a physical ability alone, but to reproduce with his body a mental image of perfect form in movement, and to gain perfect control over the execution of those movements—mental *and* physical control. The student has not learned relaxation in the face of danger, clear-mindedness, and intense concentration as *abstract* qualities to be understood only in the mind. He has trained himself to have those qualities permeate his body and become second nature to it. The mind holds an image of grace, which it teaches the body. The body has life and feeling, which it teaches the mind. Until at least the body is graceful, the mind is alive, and the two are one.

The distinction we make between mind and body in everyday speech and thought is really a matter of words and not much more. We do the same thing with all the pairs of so-called opposites: light and dark, hot and cold, male and female, spiritual and material, beauty and ugliness. All of these things are not really opposites separated by some great wall—they are degrees of some single quality, directions along a single continuum.

Take light and dark, for example. They're not two different things—they are degrees of brightness, starting from pitch black. There's no point where dark ends and light begins, right? Or take hot and cold. They're just degrees of a single quality, *heat*—starting from Absolute Zero (which is as "cold" as anything can get, 459.69° below zero Fahrenheit.) There's no line that separates hot and cold—they're just different directions along the spectrum of possible temperatures. We use the distinctions of these pairs of "opposites" because they conveniently express our perceptions of the world in a simple way—but they're not the whole truth.

That's the point about the mind and the body: For convenience we call them separate things, and think of them as opposites. But really they are only the two poles of a single entity—which is the whole person. They can never be completely separated. There's no bodily event that goes unregistered in your mind, and no mental occurrence that doesn't affect your body in some way.

All conditions of ill health are imbalances with respect to some pair of dual qualities. The cure lies in restoring balance. Here are some of the possible factors that may be involved (with explanations where necessary):

Body—Mind

Love—Fear

Flexibility—Rigidity

Nature—Culture

Affection—Hostility

Orthosympathetic—Parasympathetic

Unconscious—Conscious

The conscious mind is thought, self-consciousness, perception, virtually everything you are *aware* of. The unconscious (or subconscious) includes everything else that the mind contains: dream, memory, repressed feelings, internal perceptions of bodily functions that we are not normally aware of (such as heartbeat, action of the glands and internal organs, nervous system communications)—and possibly also such things as ESP, telepathy, clairvoyance, knowledge of past lives, psychic and spiritual phenomena of all kinds. It is possible to bring many areas of the unconscious into consciousness, such as remembering your dreams; rediscovering repressed feelings and desires through psychoanalysis or introspection; acquiring conscious control over certain functions of the autonomic nervous system by means of meditation, or biofeedback conditioning; expanding your awareness through various physical or spiritual disciplines or through other unplanned religious experiences. The unconscious mind is infinite. The capacity for integrating large areas of the unconscious into your aware waking-consciousness is a matter solely of personal development!

Spontaneous actions are those not planned or determined by the conscious mind, such as laughter; bursting into tears; orgasm; an inexplicable desire to dance, to shout, to be comforted; true compassion (which is your untaught feeling for another creature, *not* compliance with some socially-conditioned morality); anger; and often fear and violence as well. Spontaneous feelings well up from areas of the unconscious, rather than resulting from any decision of the conscious personality. The *will* is a function of the conscious mind that enables you to do something that your instincts, your body, or your unconscious would not be able to do, or would not choose to do. For example, facing an enemy who is threatening your family, *despite* an overwhelming feeling of fear, is an act of the will. Or forcing yourself to stay awake and keep moving around, shouting and singing and exercising, when you are trapped on a mountain-climbing expedition in severe cold and will suffer frostbite and maybe death if you allow yourself to rest or sleep. The will is an emergency mechanism of the human organism that can transcend all other feelings.

Some people suffer from a lack of willpower, or "weak will"—which means they can't always control their responses, even if their very survival is at stake. Other people, or even the same ones, may suffer from a lack of spontaneity. This is much more prevalent in our society. Many people show little or no spontaneity of movement, thought, or feeling. Instead, they just keep on in their often unpleasurable, deadening, painful ways of living, by means of an almost continual hold of the will. They force themselves to jobs they hate 200 or 300 days a year; they live in environments they can barely stand because they "have to"; they persist in a hundred interpersonal relationships that they don't enjoy, for one imagined necessity or another. But the will was not

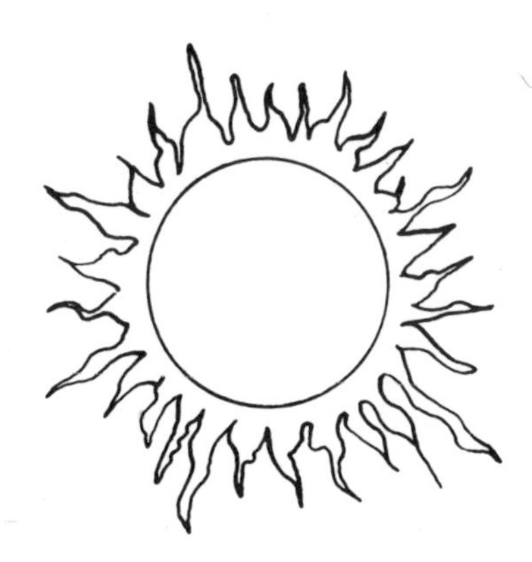

meant as a continual function of the organism, and its overuse on a long-term basis puts too great a strain on the bodymind system, continually denying or suppressing too many natural, spontaneous, instinctual feelings. Inevitably some mental, physical, or emotional disease or breakdown is bound to occur.

Aggression—Passivity ______________________________

Aggression simply means "moving toward" something —an active response. Passivity is the tendency to be still, to take no action, to do nothing. You can have aggressive hostility or aggressive affection, passive hate or passive love, any combination. Aggressiveness (like anger) is not, per se, a negative or unhealthy quality. You need a certain amount of aggressiveness as a healthy living organism—to seek out food, shelter, means of survival, a sexual mate. Only in the extreme does aggressiveness become unhealthy. The same is true of passivity, a necessary state for restoring energies and receiving information—but the extreme of which indicates some blocking or diminishing of your basic life functions.

Imagination—Realism ______________________________

We think of children as being full of imagination, experimentation, and unbridled curiosity about life—but without responsibility, without a great deal of concern for the consequences of their actions, without our "sense of reality." Adults, on the other hand, are supposed to be defined by their "realism": a knowledge of the way the world actually is, and an acceptance of the limitations that this knowledge demands. Actually, the healthy person integrates these two qualities rather than regarding them as mutually exclusive. Such a person lives, works, and functions in the "real world"—without losing the imagination, the creativity, the sense of continual discovery and wonder that most others sadly leave behind in childhood.

As you see, in every case the warring opposition of the two tendencies is a source of tension for the individual, where rightly each has its own place and natural level; finding that healthy balance is always the solution. One of the "angles" on achieving health that was mentioned before is *integrating the conscious and unconscious minds.* Here are two ways to go about this.

Dreaming

This is one experience we all share that clearly demonstrates the existence of a vast subconscious realm mostly unknown to us in our waking state. It has been proven that *all* people dream at some time during the night, but usually they remember little or nothing when they wake up. This is a good example of the lack of contact between conscious and unconscious in most people.

It *is* possible to remember your dreams more easily —by strongly telling yourself just before you go to sleep that you're going to remember them (a mild form of self-hypnosis) and by not allowing your head to immediately fill up with the days' plans and activities the minute you wake up. Forgetting is an active process, it's something getting in the way of memory—which is why people in jail, on desert islands, or living and working completely alone tend to remember their dreams much more vividly and completely. Try keeping a notebook by your bed and writing down everything you remember of your dreams each morning (even if it's only the smallest fragment), and I guarantee you'll learn a lot about yourself that you didn't know!

Meditation

What the material of dreams actually is, we don't fully know; but it's clear that there are many *other* levels of the unconscious as well, and that these also can be made conscious. Meditation is one way to do this. To meditate properly first requires *concentration*—the ability to put your attention somewhere and keep it there as long as you want. Try this concentration exercise:

Look at any object in the room (the doorknob, a lamp, a chair) and concentrate all your attention on that object, so that nothing intrudes on your awareness of it. Hold this concentration for 15 or 20 seconds. Then shift your attention to another, different object in the room (say, something small like a cup and saucer, or a pen, or an ashtray) and concentrate completely on that, again for 15 or 20 seconds. Do this with four or five different things, trying each time to eliminate *all* conscious thought except for your awareness of the single object. Then close your eyes.

With your eyes shut, concentrate on the image of the last object you looked at. Hold this image and concentrate on it as intently as if you were looking directly at it—again, for 15 or 20 seconds. Then transfer your concentration to your *feet.* Become as aware as you can of your feet, without opening your eyes—feel them, know them, concentrate on them as if nothing else existed in the world. Then switch to another part of your body (say, the top of your head) and concentrate your attention there for half a minute or so. Do this for several other parts of your body, making sure to leave the last one completely behind when you shift your attention to a new part.

Then concentrate on your hearing for a full minute. Do nothing, think nothing, just *listen.* Finally, turn your awareness to your breathing. Sit or lie in a comfortable position and feel your breathing, be conscious only of breathing. This is a good way to begin your meditation.

When your breathing has become slow, even, deep, and regular, and you are fully concentrated on it, then shift your concentration to the Hara, and keep it there for a full minute. Then gradually, gradually, *let go* of that concentration—but don't begin another. Do nothing, think nothing, *try* nothing—just be. Allow any thoughts, images, feelings, or ideas to come into your consciousness (don't try to stop them), take note of them, and let them pass on through. This is a safe, relaxed, and pleasant way to come into contact with some interesting material from your own unconscious self. But more important, it can give you a deep peace of mind and an inner tranquility that lasts. Twenty minutes of this kind of meditation every day, or whenever you feel out of touch with yourself and in need of some harmonizing, can only increase your self-understanding, clear your thinking, and help put the whole you back together. Give it a try.

The real wellsprings of life, the forces that move us most profoundly, the roots of our basic life-energies all lie deep in the unconscious. Like the iceberg whose visible part is only one-tenth of what lies beneath the surface, the everyday, conscious identity is only a fraction of the total self. Yet most people mistakenly act as if they were *only* this surface—only the little person who goes to work, who drives a car, who cooks supper, who watches television, who plays out a few roles in a few places and then sleeps.

But we are all greater beings than that. All the wisdom you need to live happily is within you already, in that nine-tenths of you beneath the surface. What you really have to do is *unlearn* the patterns that are keeping you from yourself! Cease mistrusting your nature; stop denying your body; give up seeing things only on the surface, at the level of your conscious, role-playing, socially-defined identity. There is much more to you—get back to yourself and find out!

The conscious mind *does* have many useful functions in the healthy individual, obviously. It does not have to be the enemy of the instincts, the unconscious, and the body. In the healthy balance, the head does not rule as a dictator over the body—nor the other way around. This brings us to our original question: What is your life all about? *Why* are you here on the earth? What does it mean to be alive, to have a body, to have a mind, to be a human being? Living is hard work—often painful, confusing, frightening. Why go on?

The mind alone can't answer that question. The body answers, the heart answers, the soul answers: *Life is the reason.* There is no other. Getting your mind fixed on *life* is the way of balance, the way of natural order, the way to be healthy and loving, the way to grow. Mind fixed on life. Is there anything better to have it fixed on?

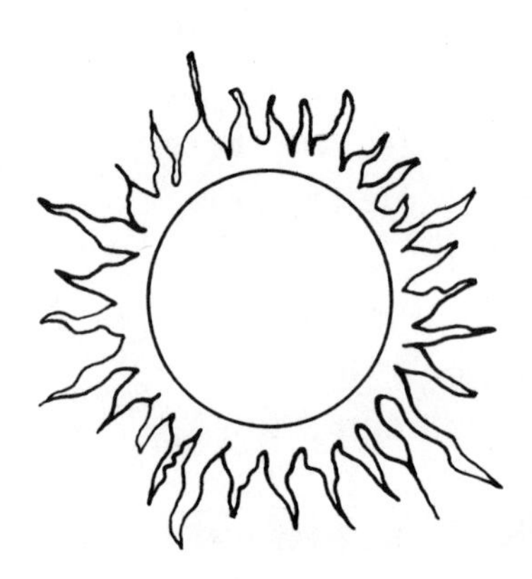

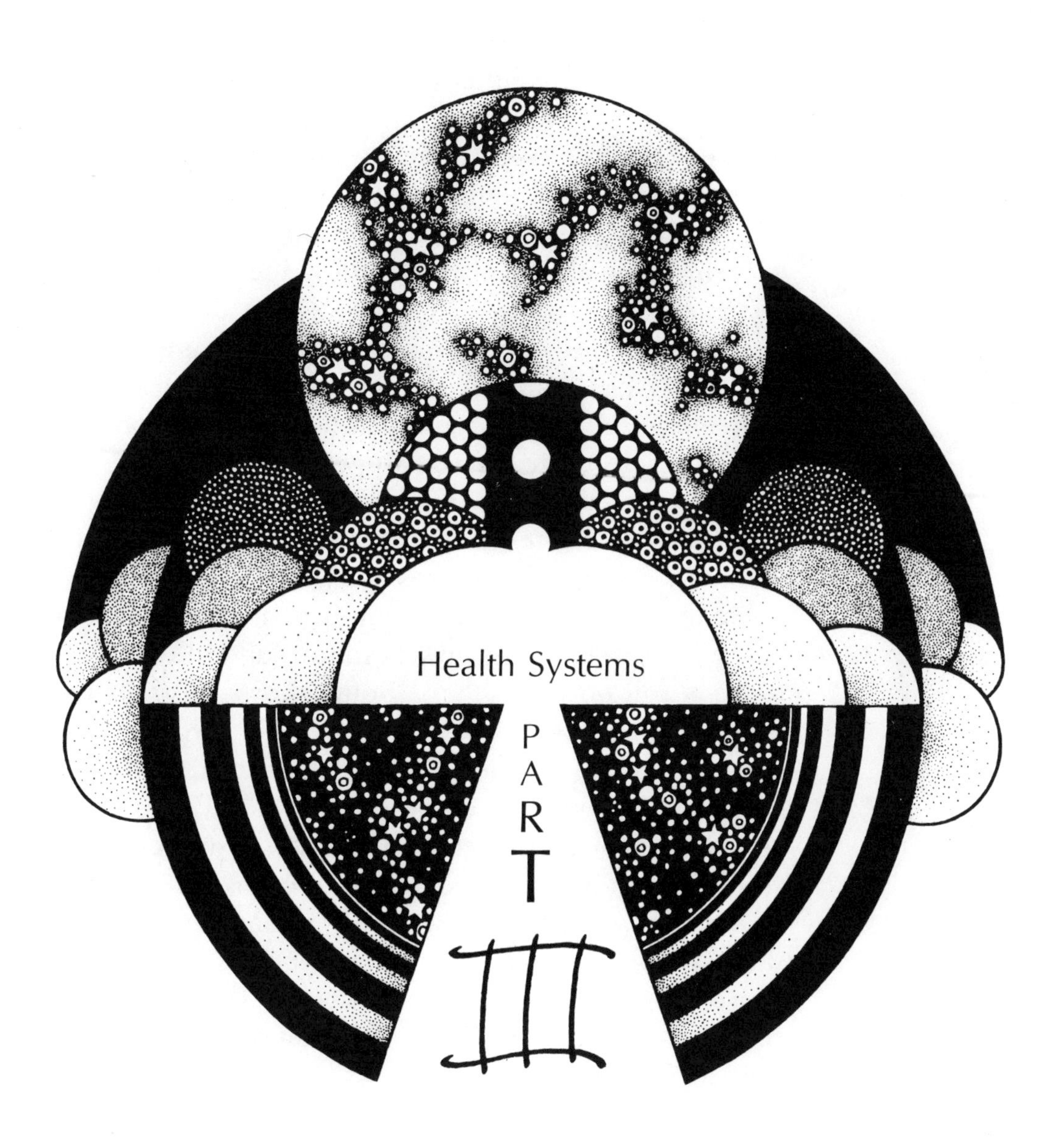
Health Systems
PART
III

Human culture is based on the noble idea that each new generation shouldn't have to learn from scratch everything that it needs to survive—but instead, inherits the wisdom, the technology, the progress (and the folly, the corruption, the crimes) of those that have gone before. Man has been scratching his head and stretching his legs for quite a long time now, and has come up with some interesting methods of mind and body development. This part of the book describes some of these systems.

The one shortcoming inherent in all systems, though, is the very fact that they *are* someone else's wisdom, someone else's science, and just as often someone else's folly. They're there for you to pick up on and start *following,* rather than hacking your own way through the wilderness of existence. My own opinion is that finding your own way is what makes you grow.

Some of the systems give you broad, clearly defined, and well-traveled highways to follow, and all you have to do is roll on down them. Some show you trails less used, going right through some beautiful woods. And some just show you how to make a fire and navigate by the stars. You may be one of those who prefers to pack your own gear and take your chances, assuming that you'll learn what you need along the way—it's a matter of personal taste. Just beware of jumping into any of the available systems so hard that you lose your *own* sense of reality and accept somebody else's view of things, on faith. And don't expect anybody to teach you how to *live.* Okay?

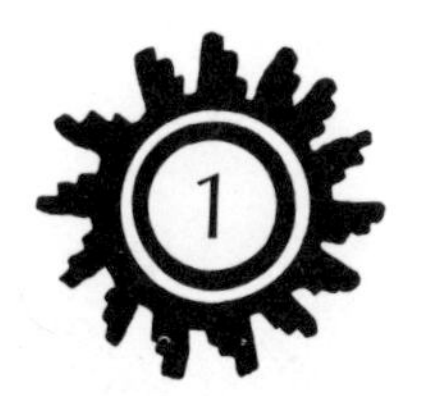

ASIAN MARTIAL ARTS

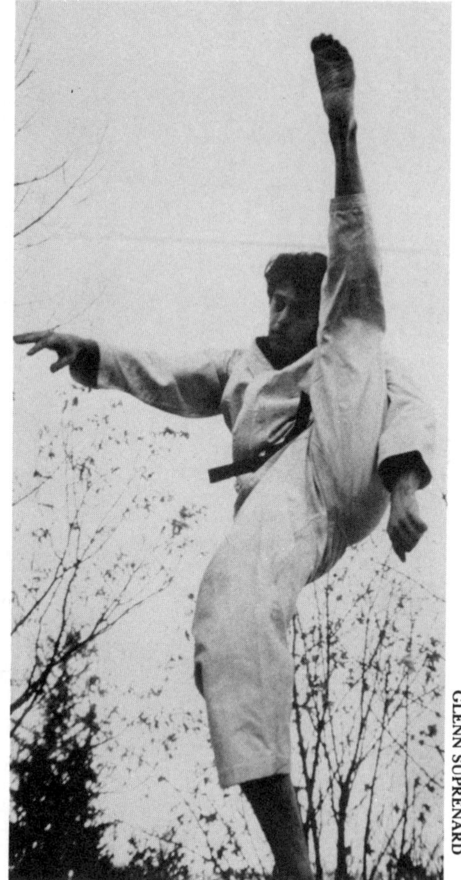

GLENN SUPRENARD

I have no parents; I make the heavens and the earth my parents.
I have no home; I make *seika tanden** my home.
I have no divine power; I make honesty my divine power.
I have no means; I make docility my means.
I have no magic power; I make personality my magic power.
I have neither life nor death; I make A UM my life and death.
I have no body; I make stoicism my body.
I have no eyes; I make the flash of lightning my eyes.
I have no ears; I make sensibility my ears.
I have no limbs; I make promptitude my limbs.
I have no laws; I make self-protection my laws.
I have no strategy; I make "free to kill and free to restore life" my strategy.
I have no designs; I make "taking opportunity by the forelock" my designs.
I have no miracles; I make righteous laws my miracles.
I have no principles; I make adaptability to all circumstances my principles.
I have no tactics; I make emptiness and fullness my tactics.
I have no talent; I make ready wit my talent.
I have no friends; I make my mind my friend.
I have no enemy; I make incautiousness my enemy.

* *Seika tanden* is the "one-point in the lower abdomen," just below the navel, considered the body's center of gravity and the center of spiritual energy; the term is in many ways synonymous with Hara.

I have no armor; I make benevolence and righteousness my armor.
I have no castle; I make immovable-mind my castle.
I have no sword; I make absence-of-mind my sword.

ANCIENT JAPANESE SAMURAI

Asian martial (fighting) arts are very ancient disciplines. They have been developed over hundreds and thousands of years as ways of uniting the body and the spirit, primarily through the laboratory of physical combat. But great ability as a fighter is not the main goal; it is the *means* by which the martial artist works to attain health of body-and-mind. The martial artist does become capable of fast and powerful movement. But more importantly, he (or she) gains clarity of mind and an unshakable inner serenity.

Judo

Today Judo is practiced all over the world as a competitive sport—it is even part of the Olympic Games competition. But in its complete form, Judo ("the gentle way") is a Jujutsu system of mind and body training that includes not only the combative techniques of throwing, falling, grappling, choking, joint-locking, and striking vital points, but also a whole lexicon of healing and resuscitation methods and the development of inner strength through meditation, breathing practice, and endless repetition of techniques. Judo training affords the benefits of aerobic exercise and develops flexibility, leg and hip strength, and self-discipline. In schools where the competitive aspects of the art are overemphasized, though, it becomes not much more than another strenuous contact sport and ceases to be a health system.

Karate

Several "empty-hand" fighting arts of Okinawa and Japan go by this name. In their classical form they are closely related to Zen philosophy, and include breathing practices, seated meditation, and a definite system of moral values—in addition to physical conditioning and the combat techniques of punching, kicking, striking, blocking, and shifting. Part of the training also includes actual sparring practice, some toughening of the "natural weapons" of hands and feet, and explicit self-defense maneuvers. Perhaps the most distinctive method of training that Karate employs is the *kata,* or form. This is a choreographed series of fighting movements, performed alone against an imaginary group of opponents. Perfection of form demands not only an excellence of movement (speed, power, accuracy, and balance) but also an intense concentration, a clear mind, and a heightened awareness. There are upwards of 50 *kata* in the various Karate styles, and their mastery represents the essential inner development of the martial artist.

The extraordinary feats of the great Karate masters—such as killing a tiger with a spear-hand thrust of the fingers, or dropping a bird in flight by the power of a shout—result from lifetimes devoted to such mind-and-body training. Great emphasis is laid on acquiring complete *control* of all movements, as well as speed and power. The true masters of the art, though, are not rigid, contained, or tense personalities; in fact, they are just the opposite. The development of such tremendous bodymind control seems to demand—or create—an equal degree of spontaneity and relaxation. Those are the qualities of real martial arts masters, who appear most unaggressive, relaxed, natural, and good-humored. Their movements appear neither strained nor forced, but effortlessly efficient.

It takes years of work to attain such a state. One Karate system, for example, Kosho-ryu Kempo, instructed its students in Buddhist philosophy, general education, the human body and its systems, fencing, archery, flower arranging, swimming, tree climbing, horsemanship, use of the blowgun, *and* weaponless combat! Needless to say, there are few schools in America that offer even a fraction of such well-rounded training. But excellent instructors *can* be found who perpetuate the spirit of mental and physical development through Budo (martial arts).

Beware of quick-karate schools, of highly aggressive or egotistical instructors, of overemphasis on competitive Karate. True Bushido (the Way of the Warrior) teaches that your only real enemy is yourself; eliminating fear is your real battle. To concentrate on beating others, especially in tournaments where other incentives such as trophies, fame, even money are introduced, works against the deeper goals of the art.

Karate training is hard, sweaty work. The movements are explosive and demand a considerable amount of bodily power. Its spiritual underpinnings, its channeling of violent energies into constructive forms, its beneficial effects on health and character make Karate—in its pure form—a highly recommended system. On the other hand, in its corrupted forms—which unfortunately are widespread these days—it can be a dangerous and destructive force. Take great care in selecting a *dojo* (school) and *sensei* (teacher).

Here is a breathing exercise from Japanese Karate: Stand straight, with your hands in front of your waist, you fists closed. Concentrate you attention on the Hara, which should be lightly tensed. Inhale deeply and slowly through your nostrils, filling your abdomen, rib cage, and chest with breath as you bring your arms circularly up and out in front of you, the fists crossing each other in front of your chest. Complete the inhale with hands raised above your head and spread wide apart—this coordination of the hands and the breath is important. You should be gazing slightly upwards at this time. Hold this position for a few seconds only, but feel the breath you have taken in filling your whole body, right down to your feet. Don't lose your concentration on Hara. Exhale slowly, through your mouth, tensing your abdomen and forcing the air through your tensed throat with a deep "haaa" sound. At the same time bring your fists down, circularly again, to the starting point, hands still tightly clenched. Press every last ounce of air out of your lungs, looking straight ahead. Repeat this whole cycle three times in all, then relax. This exercise is good for catching your breath when winded, clearing impurities from your lungs, concentrating your spirit, and unifying mind and body.

Korean Karate (includes Tae Kwon Do, Tang Soo Do, Hapkido, Hwarang Do, Tae Gyun)

Korean Karate is similar to the Japanese and Okinawan systems, but the style of movement is somewhat more circular and relaxed. Korea occupies a geographical and cultural position midway between Japan and China—and the Korean martial arts are a unique synthesis of the "hard" Okinawan-Japanese tendency and the "soft" Chinese tendency. In Korean styles the legs are the main weapons rather than the hands. Expert Korean martial artists are renowned for their fast and incredibly powerful high side kicks, roundhouse kicks, and jumping techniques.

This emphasis on the legs makes Korean Karate an extremely strong fighting form—and also an excellent way of restoring body balance in "overcivilized" people who sit most of the day, drive cars rather than walk or run, and channel all their energy upwards, weakening

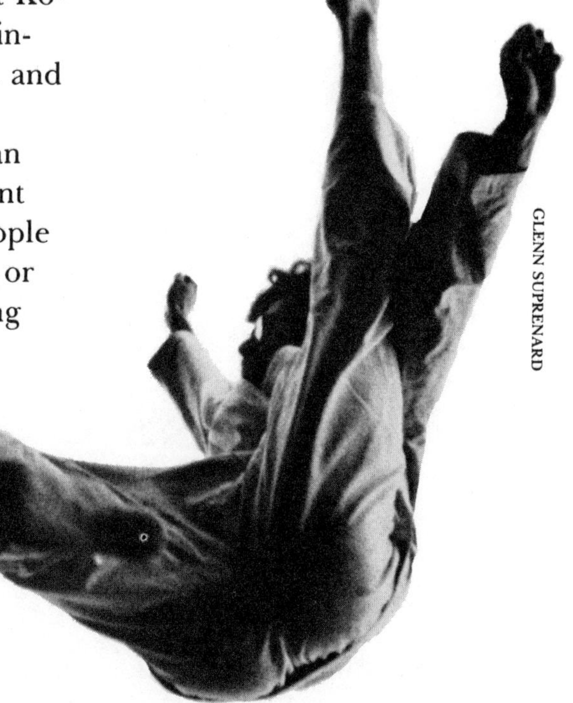

GLENN SUPRENARD

the lower body. Through the practice of Korean Karate the hips become more flexible, the legs strengthen and become more "conscious," the feet and ankles come *alive.*

Korean Karate is rapidly becoming the most popular style in the United States; and the same precautions apply that I mentioned above. There are, however, excellent instructors to be found. Properly taught and properly studied, Korean Karate develops stillness of mind, nonaggression, a graceful and powerful use of energy, harmony, and good health.

A good practice to get just a little of the feeling of the leg-energy used in Korean Karate is to stand in Horse Stance: feet parallel and wide apart (about two shoulder widths), with your knees well bent and bowed out—as if you were riding a horse. Keep your shoulders relaxed; your spine straight; your hips directly below your shoulders, neither tucked in nor pushed back. In this position you should feel the weight of your upper body sunk down to your hips, feel the solidity and balance of your stance, feel power and strength in your feet, legs, and hips. Holding this Horse Stance, do the Karate breathing exercise described earlier. Then try stepping and shifting to different directions, keeping you body low and maintaining the Horse Stance each time. Do this for five full minutes without once straightening your legs and you'll be *much* more aware of your legs!

Kung Fu

The name Kung Fu applies to an astonishingly wide variety of Chinese combat and development systems. Technically, some emphasize flowery, circular hand techniques; some specialize in footwork; others teach the striking of vital points with the fingertips, or the more occult possibilities like delayed-action "death touches" and the use of psychic powers. The Chinese arts are marked by their fluid, circular movements, which appear deceptively "soft." Many of the stances and techniques are based on animal movement patterns—such as the Crane Stance, the Tiger Claw, the Praying Mantis Style, and so on. Mental and spiritual training is at least as important as technique in the true Kung Fu.

Many Chinese systems also include medicinal techniques and healing, uses of special weapons, and knowledge of nerve centers. They work on developing some of the more interesting capabilities of the human animal. For example, Alan Lee, a New York Wu Shu instructor, gives public demonstrations in which he stops his heartbeat (as measured by electrodes taped to his body) and then starts it again at will! Lee has also demonstrated his powers of "internal resistance" publicly (on a nationwide TV show) by lying on a bed of sharp nails with a 500-pound slab of stone on top of him, which is then smashed to pieces by an assistant wielding a sledgehammer.

Kung Fu, and in fact any martial art, is nothing to be taken up lightly. Until only a few years ago Kung Fu was not taught publicly, nor even privately, to non-Chinese. The situation is now changing and several *kwoon* (clubs) with excellent instructors have opened their doors.

These four systems are the best-known of the major "external" schools of Asian unarmed martial arts. They apply the concentration of muscular energy to develop speed, power, and coordination. Over a long period of time, through endless repetition of techniques, regular practice of *forms* (the dancelike prearranged combat movement patterns), breathing exercises, meditation, and sparring, a higher level of relaxed and graceful (yet even more powerful) movement is attained—together with a certain psychological transformation. They are serious undertakings, but well worth the effort.

> Boxing requires movement,
> but first, the Internal requires stillness;
> To defeat the enemy requires strength,
> but first, the Internal requires softness;
> Fighting requires speed,
> but first, the Internal requires slowness.
>
> PA KUA SAYING

The Oriental symbol for the continuous interplay of apparent opposites (light and dark, active and passive, etc.) is the T'ai Chi. This literally means the "Grand Ultimate," and refers to the great Unity that lies behind all polarities and is the true order of the universe—or Tao.

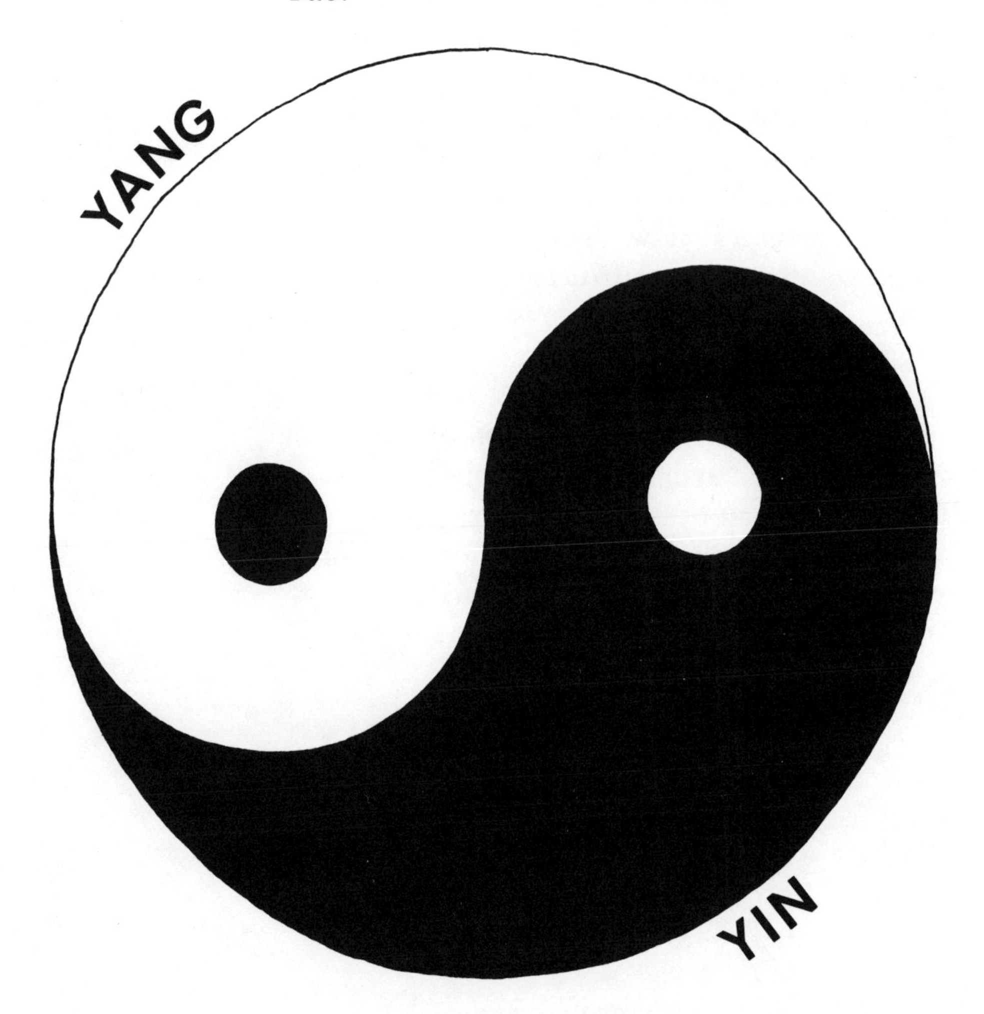

The dark aspect is called *Yin,* and refers to the "female" principle—the receptive, the downward, the earthly, the soft, the yielding. The light aspect is called *Yang,* and refers to the "male" principle—the giving, the upward-moving, the sun, the sky, the strong, the unyielding, the rigid, the hard. Within the circle of the martial arts, the "External" schools can be considered Yang (although some are certainly softer than others—notably the Chinese styles), and the "Internal" schools, Yin.

The Internal schools do not rely on sheer muscular force and coordination for their source of power and combat effectiveness. They rely on ki (Japanese) or ch'i (Chinese)—your "intrinsic" or inner energy—which is something other than physical in origin. Students of the Internal schools devote even more attention than those of the External to cultivation of the spirit, calming the mind and directing its concentrated attention, and unifying the self in a harmonious, graceful whole.

The Internal arts do not require a great deal of physical strength, and there is less apparent violence in the movements themselves. They tend to be preferred over the External by women and older people. (As self-defense systems, however, they are by no means inferior; in fact, the opposite is true.) Essentially, though, the choice of a martial art depends on your character—not your age, sex, or physical development. Only two of the existing Internal martial arts are practiced widely in the West: T'ai Chi Ch'uan and Aikido.

T'ai Chi Ch'uan

Millions of Chinese, on the Mainland and elsewhere around the globe, can be seen every day at sunrise and sunset, in the courtyards and the playgrounds and the fields, performing the long, graceful, slow-motion dancelike pattern of movements that is the elemental practice of T'ai Chi. The essence of this practice is relaxation-in-movement.

As you go through the long form, you strive to keep your weight sunk to the navel region, your breathing slow and even and from the belly, your mind calm and tranquil, and your every movement graceful and continuous, "like pulling silk from a cocoon." There is no muscular tension anywhere, yet your spine is straight, as if you were suspended from above. Your movements are fluid and natural—yet they are precise.

> The energy is rooted in the feet, develops in the legs, is directed by the waist, and functions through the fingers. The feet, the legs, and the waist act as one whole unit. . . .
>
> FROM THE *T'ai Chi Ch'uan Classics,* BY CHANG SAN-FENG OF THE WUTANG MOUNTAIN, 13TH CENTURY A.D.

This formal practice alone, done twice a day for 15 to 20 minutes, is capable of improving your health remarkably. It makes your breathing deeper and slower, and promotes better circulation of the blood. Your internal organs receive a gentle massage and their functioning gradually improves. The movements of your body become relaxed, graceful, and centered in the waist region. And, most significantly, your entire character can be altered, as mental conflicts and emotional tensions are dissolved in the gently flowing river of the T'ai Chi form.

The explanation for all this is ch'i. The flow of ch'i throughout your body, stimulated by correct practice and abdominal breathing, benefits all the life functions. The Chinese call ch'i the "spirit of vitality" or "tenacious energy"; a Western scientist might call it the "psychophysiological power associated with blood and breath." It has many explanations and many interpretations—but ch'i is real, and its effects are often astounding. T'ai Chi masters have attained the ability to be struck with sledgehammers and not be hurt; to uproot and send flying opponents twice their size with a gentle, effortless movement; even to repulse an attack from behind before it has reached their body—all through the cultivation of ch'i.

> Chinese say that whoever practices T'ai Chi, correctly and regularly, twice a day over a period of time, will gain the pliability of a child, the health of a lumberjack, and the peace of mind of a sage.
>
> CHENG MAN CHING, *T'ai Chi*

T'ai Chi can be practiced for health purposes only—as it is by millions of people around the world, of all ages and sexes. But the principles of the art can also be applied to combat, in the form of T'ai Chi Ch'uan (*ch'uan* means "fist")—an apparently soft yet devastatingly fast and powerful fighting system.

Aikido

"Aikido holds that all bodily movements must agree with the laws of nature." It is a fluid, circular, effortless-looking yet tremendously potent martial art, based upon the cultivation of *ki.* The art was developed by Morihei Uyeshiba, one of the most amazing men to have lived in this century.

Uyeshiba had built himself up from a sickly youth into one of the strongest Jujutsu fighters and swordsmen in all Japan. But the discord and the hatred in the world troubled him, and while at the peak of his physical prowess he went into the mountains to meditate. He lived alone in a small cabin for five years. One day he

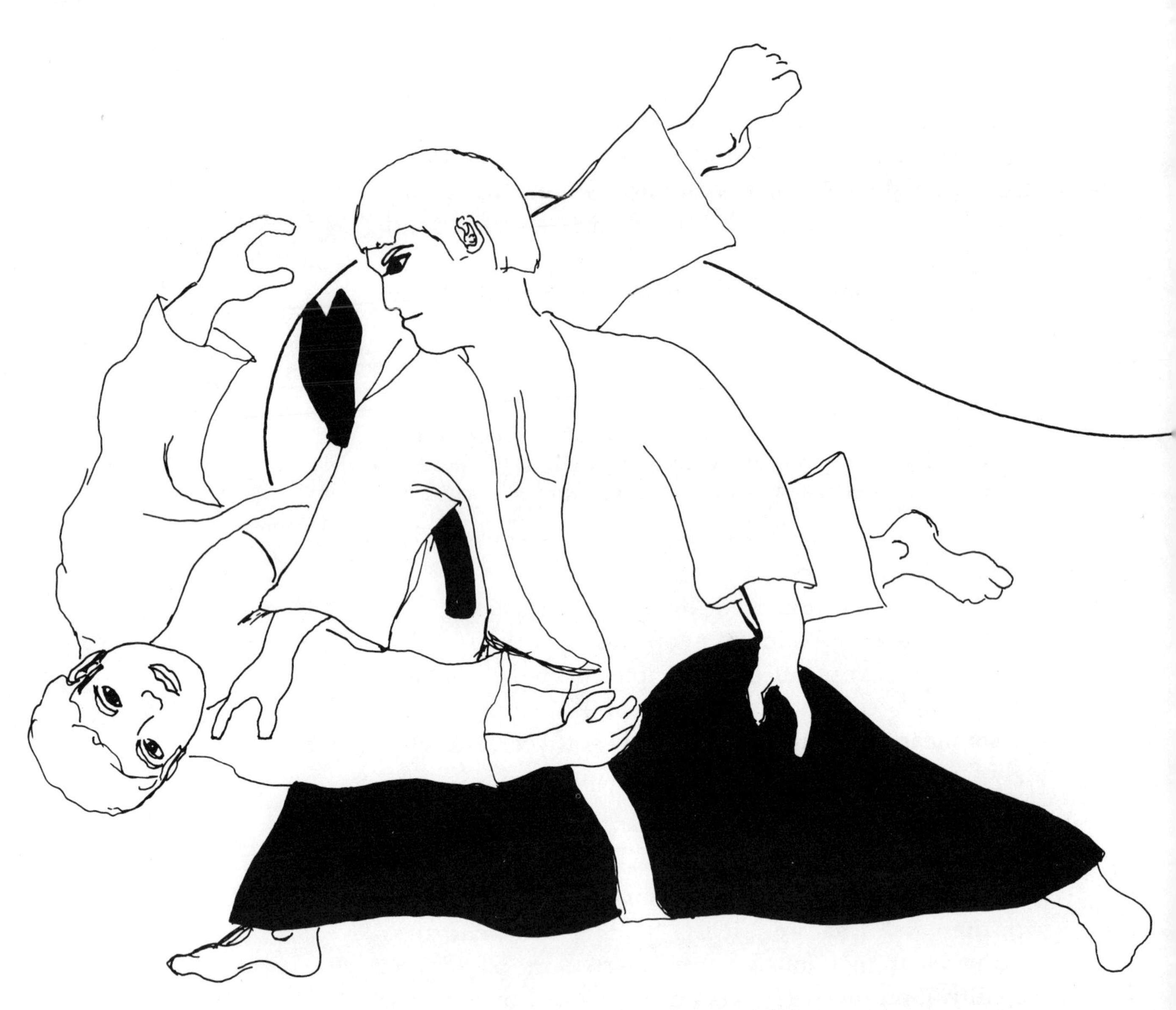

decided to return to the world of men. Stopping in a garden to refresh himself by showering water over his body, Uyeshiba looked up into the blue sky—and was suddenly enlightened. He was rooted to the ground. "All he felt was joy; all he knew was gratitude to the Universal. Suddenly, he saw the heart of the universe . . . he perceived his own oneness with the universe." He was filled with a radiant life-energy, which he called *ki*. He said, "The martial arts are love!"

Uyeshiba spent the rest of his life developing and teaching Aikido, which means "the way to harmony with ki." Even in his eighties he was unbelievably agile, fast, graceful, relaxed, radiant, and powerful. He was observed, even by the most skeptical of critics, to have defeated high-ranking young Karate experts and other trained martial artists with such speed and dexterity that they could not say how he had thrown them, or even where they had been touched! In the late 1960s, a friend of mine saw him give a demonstration at Boston University. Uyeshiba supported a 250-pound football player hanging on the *wrist* of his outstretched arm—with no visible strain or effort on his part, and his arm muscles completely relaxed. Uyeshiba was past 80, and weighed about 120 pounds at the time. This was a small demonstration of the power of ki.

He died in 1969, leaving Aikido, a physical-spiritual discipline that would enable those who practiced it sincerely to achieve:

1. Superb physical health
2. An efficient yet nonaggressive means of self-defense (Aikido uses no striking or kicking techniques)
3. The unification of body and spirit
4. The reconstruction of human society, based upon higher principles

Ultimately, Uyeshiba said, "It is the way to reconcile the world and make human beings one family."

How do Aikidoists explain the force of Ki? "Aikido refers to the forces behind all things as Ki. . . . Ki is the elemental basis of the universe. Call it God or call it Buddha, it is still the same. Only the method of explaining it and the disciplines vary." (Koichi Tohei) Ki is the universal spirit as it moves in your own bodymind. But training and strengthening the body alone is not enough:

> The truth is that only those who strive to train their spirits as well as their bodies turn out to be men of the highest caliber. . . . As long as the person is young and healthy, his spirit too remains in good condition; but . . . with advancing years and the afflictions of illness, his spirit tends to weaken. . . . Yet this is the very time when a strong and tenacious spirit is essential. The spirit need not be ill just because the body is. . . . The strong spirit is that which does not falter in adversity and which is not moved in time of trouble. . . . Aikido always concentrates on a study of the rules of the spirit—that is, on the rules of ki. Our discipline is focused on discovering how giving full play to the rules of the spirit can favorably affect the body.
>
> WESTBROOK AND RATTI,
> *Aikido and the Dynamic Sphere*

Here is an example of applied ki, which you can try: Stand normally. Tense your muscles, swell your chest, think of directing your energy upwards. Have a friend put his arms around your chest and lift you off the ground. You should be fairly easy to lift. (If not, find a stronger friend!)

Then relax all your muscles—especially your shoulders, back, chest, buttocks, and thighs. Bend your knees slightly, breathe from the abdomen, and feel your *feet* in contact with the ground. Feel your energy flowing downwards, connecting you to the earth, as if your legs had roots. Now have your friend try to lift you, in the same way.

You will have become much "heavier," and if your concentration is particularly good, he won't be able to lift you off the ground at all. Although your body hasn't moved, and it still weighs exactly the same, your ki has changed direction—and "you" are not the same. Aikido practitioners can become so well-rooted to the ground this way that three or four strong men can't even budge them. (I've seen this demonstration myself more than once and can vouch for it.)

You can feel the flow of ki in another way: Stand or sit quietly with your eyes closed. Relax. Concentrate all your attention into the index finger of one hand; close the other fingers lightly into a fist. Imagine a radiant energy, like a warm, glowing liquid, flowing down through your arm and out from the fingertip and a thousand miles beyond. In a short while you'll begin to feel a tingling sensation in the fingertip, and it may start to feel warm. This is the beginning of the flow of ki.

"Martial Arts," said one of my teachers, "are the creation of individual myth." Properly taught and diligently practiced, they can become the basis for a very healthy way of life. At some point every student finally leaves his or her master and becomes an independent and unique "system"—for the goal of these exacting and highly structured disciplines is not obedience, but liberation.

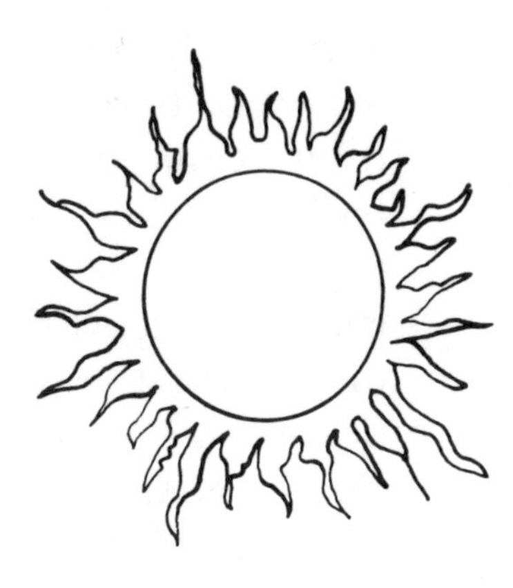

YOGA

Yoga is a spiritual discipline that works toward the attainment of union (*yoga* in Sanskrit) of the Individual Self (Atman) with the Infinite Self (Brahman). Yoga is ancient, perhaps 5,000 years old, and it contains a vast array of information about the human being and his or her potential development, particularly in terms of spiritual consciousness.

There are many types of Yoga, all of which represent different possible routes to the same goal—union of man with the so-called Ultimate Reality. The main forms are: Bhakti Yoga, the Yoga of devotional love; Jnana Yoga, the Yoga of study; Raja Yoga, the Yoga of consciousness; Hatha Yoga, the Yoga of physical health; Kundalini Yoga, the Yoga of spinal energy; Mantra Yoga, the Yoga of chanting and sounds; and Karma Yoga, the Yoga of work and action. Many of these systems tend to draw the practitioner *away* from worldly reality, from the troubles of living, and from human interaction. They do this not merely as a temporary engagement in a "separate reality" for the purpose of gaining some wisdom or powers of the soul that may then be used to regenerate the world, but often as a permanent, "other-wordly" way of life. For this reason I'm not going to treat them here as health systems—with one exception.

That exception is Hatha Yoga, an amazingly extensive science of the physical body (*and* its perfection as a means of spiritual development), which is probably one of the most important health systems ever developed by man.

"Hatha" is like Yang-Yin. "Ha" means the flow of positive energy; "Tha" means the conservation of energy, or negative energy. Ha means Sun, Tha means Moon. Hatha Yoga is a unique system of psychophysical development by means of *Asanas* (postures), *Pranayama* (breathing practices), and associated exercises *(Mudras),* controls *(Bandhas),* and purifications.

> The path to be followed is that of making our body and all its activities conscious. Even the sympathetic nervous system and all those organs whose functioning is usually independent of my consciousness can be made subservient to my will. The incalculable advantage of this is that any malfunctioning can be prevented, and the body saved from diseases which originate in functional causes. The Hatha Yogi who has reached the highest level has complete and absolute control over his body. . . . The law of the spirit is selflessness, whereas that of the body is selfishness. And yet man must learn to join the two in complete harmony and manifest them in himself. This truth was taught by all prophets and great teachers who ever lived on earth, for they knew the secret of being: the tension between the positive and negative pole. . . . The positive pole is in the top of the skull, at the spot where our hair forms a whorl. . . . The negative pole is in the coccyx, the lowest vertebra. Between these poles there is a current of extremely high frequency and short wavelength. This tension is LIFE! The carrier of life is the spinal column.
>
> YESUDIAN AND HAICH,
> *Yoga and Health*

Yogic asanas are positions of the body, slowly stretched into and held—usually coordinated with controlled breathing. Some examples are: the Lotus position (the classic meditation pose), the Yoga Headstand, the Cobra, and the Plough. Many of the asanas are concerned with bending, twisting, and flexing the spine so as to free the flow of electrical nerve-energy. Others are designed primarily to stimulate and balance the secretions of the ductless glandular system—including the thyroid, pituitary, pineal, suprarenal, and sexual glands. (These glands, as Western science now acknowledges, are the body's internal chemists, doctors, medicine men and magicians. Their secretions into the bloodstream affect your physical and emotional condition perhaps more than any other factor!)

Still other asanas are designed to stretch, loosen, relax, and strengthen various muscles and joints of the body—especially those that are chronically tense or weak, like the neck and face muscles, shoulders, hips, and small of back. Other Yoga exercises give massaging effects to the internal organs not normally affected by Western-type activities: the liver, kidneys, pancreas, spleen. And of course many asanas combine their effects on several of these aspects of the body, coordinated by a concentrated directing of the mind.

Here's a pair of Hatha Yoga asanas you can try (and their therapeutic effects as described by Selvarajan Yesudian and Elisabeth Haich):

Halasana (the Plough) • Lie down on your back, on a cloth or a blanket, with your arms alongside your body and your palms down. Relax. Exhale. Now slowly lift your feet off the gound, continuing to raise them until they're over your head. Keeping your back as relaxed as possible, your palms still on the floor, allow your feet to continue over until—if you can make it without straining—your toes touch the floor. (You can bend your knees to help you accomplish this.) Relax, and breathe

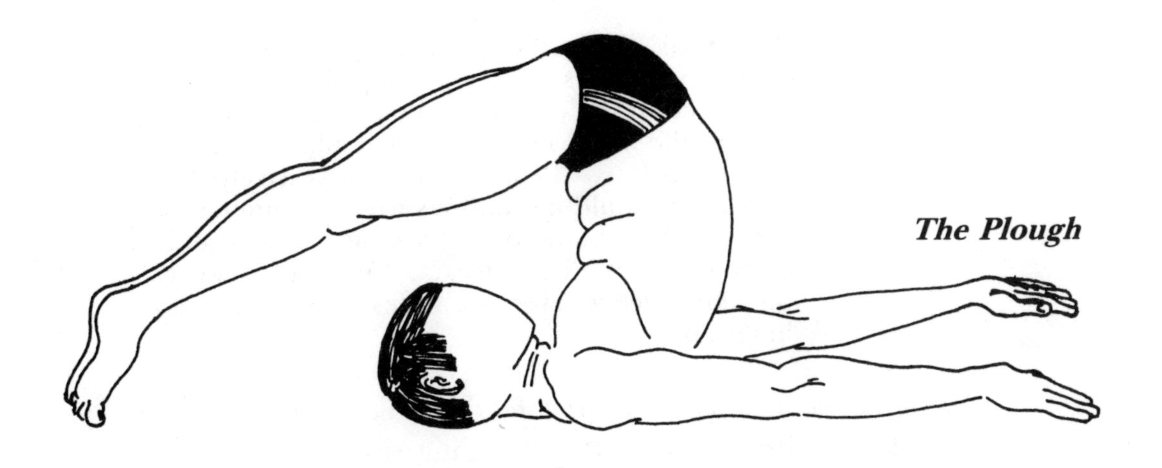

The Plough

deeply in this position three or four times. Then try to push your feet even further out away from your head, gradually straightening your legs and shifting your body weight higher up toward the top of your spine. At this point you can put both hands under your neck, or keep them on the floor, or stretch your arms back so that your toes are resting in your upturned palms—try all three variations, in fact. Stay in the most extreme position that you can hold *comfortably* for at least three or four more long, deep breaths. Then slowly unroll and let your legs down, until you are lying flat again. Breathe, and relax. Yesudian and Haich say:

> This splendid exercise not only benefits the nerves of the spinal column but also the vertebrae themselves. Persons whose vertebrae have been pulled out of position through a sedentary way of life can restore their spine to normal by means of this posture. . . . Body symmetry is enhanced to the point of perfection, and simultaneously the production of negative and positive currents is balanced. The tensing and flexing of the back muscles has a regenerating and strengthening effect on them. The organs of the abdominal cavity are tightly compressed and their blood supply increased. This exercise has a rejuvenating effect on

> the sexual glands, the pancreas, liver, spleen, and suprarenal glands. This asana also has a strengthening effect on the organs of the thorax and the region of the neck. The entire glandular system is rejuvenated. . . . People with an excessively stiff backbone should be cautious when beginning this exercise. We should bend backwards slowly and cautiously, not all at once. . . . With a few weeks' diligent practice, even the stiffest spine begins to limber up.

Dhanurasana (the Bow) • Lie face down on a rug, cloth, or blanket. Relax completely. Inhaling slowly, arch your back, bend your knees, and grab your ankles with your hands. Keep your knees pretty close together, lift your legs and head up, and arch your back as much as you can without it becoming painful. Hold this position through several breath cycles, rocking backwards and forwards a little. Then *slowly* release your ankles, and exhale as you return your legs, chest, arms, and head to the floor. Relax again. Yesudian and Haich say:

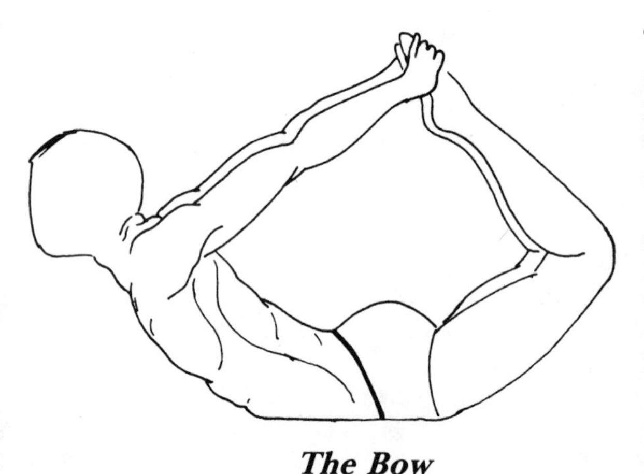

The Bow

> This exercise has a highly stimulating effect on the endocrine glands. Starting with the thyroid, it affects the thymus, hilum, liver, kidneys, suprarenal capsule, pancreas, and especially sexual glands, strengthening them and increasing their activity. . . . The entire spinal column and all nerve centers are strengthened, and their resilience preserved. Both the stimulating effect on glandular activity and the tensing and contraction of the muscles tend to prevent accumulations of fat. . . . Dhanurasana should *not* be performed in cases of hyper-function of the thyroid or excessive growth of any of the other ductless glands. The exercise should be begun very cautiously, and only little by little should we increase the length of time we hold the posture. The solar plexus is recharged with vital force.

Pranayama consists of breathing exercises designed to increase the body's store of prana. As I stated earlier, prana is the same as ki or ch'i: the elemental energy of the universe. Prana is in all substances, but it is not those substances. In man it is manifest as vitality, physical or mental energy—the spirit of life itself. Prana is most accessible to man, the Yogic science claims, from the air, through proper breathing.

Pranayama breathing exercises also increase the supply of *oxygen* to your bloodstream, and are valuable for this reason alone. Breathing practice, as mentioned earlier, is especially necessary for sedentary city-dwellers, whose shallow breathing habits over the years have greatly diminished their vitality—and whose lungs are filled with the poisons of foul air, industrial pollution, automobile exhaust, cigarette smoke, dust, and whatever else comes floating their way from out of the hazy urban skies. The two most basic pranayama are Complete Yoga Breathing (already outlined in Part II, Chapter Two) and Alternate Nostril Breathing.

Alternate Nostril Breathing

This is a great exercise for regaining your peace of mind, quieting your troubled nerves, and general psychosomatic balancing. First, make sure both nostrils are clear. Exhale completely. Place the tip of the index finger of your right hand (southpaws can reverse all these directions) at the point between your eyebrows; close your right nostril with your thumb and slowly inhale through your left nostril for a count of eight. Then hold your breath for a count of eight. Close your left nostril with your third finger and exhale through your right nostril for a count of eight. Pause for just a second after exhaling, then switch directions: Inhale through the right nostril, keeping your third finger on the left; hold for eight; exhale through the left nostril, closing the right one with your thumb. This is one complete Alternate Breathing Cycle—in through left, hold, out through right; pause; in through right, hold, out through left. Repeat three complete cycles, then stop. After you have become comfortable doing this exercise, you can change the rhythm to 4-count inhale, 16-count hold, 8-count exhale; or to whatever other rhythm feels best for you. Practice this breathing exercise often—its benefits are great.

You probably noticed during this exercise that at least one of your nostrils was not completely clear, but was blocked by mucus or some other foreign matter that shouldn't be there. In the course of living we inevitably take toxic or just plain unwanted substances into our bodies—through the air, food, and drink that we consume. Also, the body itself produces many waste products that become dangerous if they are not promptly eliminated. Hatha Yoga devotes a great deal of attention to various cleansing practices, which are mainly concerned with *internal* cleansing.

Most of these are not advisable to attempt without competent supervision; but there is one simple cleansing of the nasal passages that almost anyone can do. Here it is:

Close one nostril and sniff a small amount (a teaspoonful is fine) of warm, salted water up the other nostril. Expel it vigorously in a snorting action. Repeat this several times, alternating nostrils. While this is discomforting to most people the first time they try it, it's a very good way of preventing a bad cold from developing. It keeps your nostrils and nasal passages clean and free of obstructions, helping you avoid the unhealthy practice of mouth-breathing. And it may actually carry out accumulated waste matter that has been plugging up your sinuses for years! Incidentally, this Yogic cleansing practice is also an old European folk remedy. Complete deep breathing through clear, open nasal passages is one of the great joys of life—try it and see!

For a full experience of the Hatha Yoga system, you should properly study it under a competent instructor—preferably a *guru,* or master. But most people don't have the opportunity to do this. There is a great deal of Hatha Yoga that can be learned and practiced alone. *Yoga and Health,* by Yesudian and Haich, and *Yoga for Americans,* by Indra Devi, are two excellent books that will serve as a good introduction to the Hatha Yoga system.

MUSCLES, SPORTS, AND EXERCISES

Many Americans engage in competitive sports, calisthenics, isometrics, weight training, and so on, for their health. Some of the disadvantages of these activities as health-improvers are:

1. They tend to develop the external muscles without benefiting the internal organs (lungs, heart, kidneys, for example) correspondingly.
2. They don't necessarily unify body and mind, and may even exaggerate the separation.
3. They are usually not integrated into the larger scheme of the person's way of life, but are kept separate from it and taken up as a recreation—or an unpleasant chore.
4. In some cases the physical benefits are one-sided or imbalanced some other way (for example, tennis develops strength and coordination in your racket-wielding arm, but not the other side).

Nonetheless, there are lots of good reasons to pursue these activities. Certain areas of your body that may be particularly weak can be developed—for example, someone with very weak legs relative to his total body weight might benefit a great deal from a careful program of weight lifting to develop his thigh, buttock, calf, and foot muscles. Also, the enthusiasm and enjoyment that lots of us take in these kinds of sports and exercises may bring out more spontaneous, healthy energy than any effort of the will could summon. Finally, *any* vigorous use of your body, no matter what it is, makes you more conscious of your health and your physical-mental condition. Activity makes you *want* to move more, become more skillful, more graceful, more energetic —and nothing should be said against that!

Weight Training

Weight training, or weight lifting, is any developing of physical strength by manipulating heavy objects (usually barbells and dumbbells) so as to tax the muscles involved to such a degree that they grow in size and increase their capacity to do work. This takes place as the muscle fibers become thicker and the number of capillaries increases, providing better transportation of oxygen and nutrients to the muscle, and better removal of wastes (carbon dioxide, lactic acid) from the muscle. Physical energy is set free in the muscles themselves by the oxidation of foodstuffs brought there by the blood.

There are many specific weight-training exercises, which I'm not going to go into here; but there are a few pertinent distinctions that should be made among them. There are exercises that use only one particular set of muscles; others use more of the whole body musculature, working as a unit. An example of the first kind is the Bench Press (lying on your back, you press a weight from your chest by straightening your arms), which involves only the tricep muscles of the upper arm and the pectoral (chest) muscles. An example of the second kind is the Snatch (lifting a bar from the floor to the overhead position in one motion, by raising your back and lifting your arms while dropping one leg backwards and bending the other), which employs the thighs, calves, back, shoulders, biceps, triceps, forearms, buttocks, and neck muscles!

Obviously, this second type of exercise is much better for your overall body condition; also, these exercises are more graceful and less prone to create muscle imbalances. Many exercises, in fact, can be modified to involve more muscles by "cheating"—that is, throwing your body to assist the lift. A good example of cheating could be the Curl (raising the bar from thighs to shoulders, with your palms turned up), which normally uses only the biceps and forearms, but by cheating involves the stomach, legs, buttocks, chest, and shoulders as well.

Second distinction: high and low "reps." "Reps" are repetitions—the number of times a particular exercise is repeated within each set before stopping. High reps (10 or more) with relatively lighter weights improve muscular endurance, speed, and definition. Low reps (sometimes as few as one or two in a set) with heavier weights increase power and bulk, although they *may* reduce speed and mobility. Low reps with very heavy weights also involve the danger of straining muscles, tendons, and ligaments that cannot accommodate the great stress —especially around the knees, elbows, and back.

Weight training is an appropriate exercise form for the very limited purpose of strengthening the external muscles. Too often, though, this outward appearance of strength is equated with a state of total health—which it is not. As an adjunct or a partial component of a complete health program, weight training *can* be useful, especially in rebalancing body proportions and repairing muscles atrophied from disease or disuse.

Isometrics

Isometric contraction is similar to weight training in that it is concerned only with the external musculature. However, it's even one step further removed from any resemblance to natural body mobility, in that it involves absolutely no movement at all! The muscles to be trained isometrically are contracted against an immovable object (such as a door jamb) or against another set of muscles pulling antagonistically.

Example:

Clasp your hands together in front of you, one palm up, the other down. Push them hard against each other. You'll feel the tricep muscle (outside of the upper arm) tensing in the downward-pushing arm—and the bicep muscle (inside of the upper arm) tensing in the upward-pulling arm. If you keep up this pressing, hard, for six seconds, then switch hands, and repeat that three times (both ways), then you have "worked out" your arms isometrically!

Note that no part of your body has *moved;* that your breathing has not increased or deepened significantly; your heart is not pounding; your circulation has not been improved, except for the blood that rushes back into your upper arms after the contraction; and your sense of yourself as an organic mental-physical unity has not particularly been called forth.

Again, there *is* a limited usefulness for isometric exercise:

1. When dynamic movement is not possible—as for the bedridden or otherwise confined person
2. When the development of a specific muscle or set of muscles is desired in a very short space of time—preferably as a supplement to some more rounded routine
3. As a practice in body awareness, making you able to direct your attention to, and activate, any muscle in your body. This is a good way to discover hidden tensions in your body, to relax, even to get to sleep when you're having trouble sleeping.

Example:

Lie down and, starting with your feet, slowly work up your entire body, tensing every muscle and its antagonist, then relaxing them completely. (Muscles come in rough pairs, like bicep and tricep, that contract in opposite directions; so, if you contract both muscles in a pair at the same time, they'll both be working, even straining, although absolutely no movement occurs.) Tense and relax your toes, arches, ankle flexors, calves, thighs (front and back), buttocks, stomach and abdomen, back (lower, middle, and upper), chest, lats (outside of upper back), shoulders, arms, forearms, hands, neck, face, scalp. If you find places that are already tense, tense them a bit more and then relax them. Become aware of your whole muscular-skeletal structure and how it works. Feel the muscles beneath your skin, and the bones beneath your muscles. From this kind of isometric contraction-and-relaxation, designed for awareness and not for strength, you can become able to tense or relax any part of your body at will. Then you can isolate problems of tension or weakness when they occur and be able to direct energy to any part of you, either statically (producing tension) or dynamically (producing motion).

Calisthenics

These are exercises to increase strength, flexibility, and coordination, using no apparatus and no weight other than the body itself. Calisthenic exercise can hardly be called a health system in and of itself—it doesn't benefit the heart and lungs significantly, lacks the motivating factors of a sport or some other art where a particular grace or skill can be acquired, and seems prone to being undertaken mechanically, without any underlying mental concentration or emotional force. (How deeply involved can you get with push-ups and sit-ups?)

Still, simple calisthenic body movements form a part of many other more involving regimes—as stretching and warming-up exercises, and for developing certain muscles and certain movement patterns. It is possible to get some pretty complex and very strenuous types of movement in calisthenic practice, some of which begin to border on gymnastics. The repetition of certain of these more interesting exercises can have definitely positive effects of your physical condition and your overall health. Here are two examples:

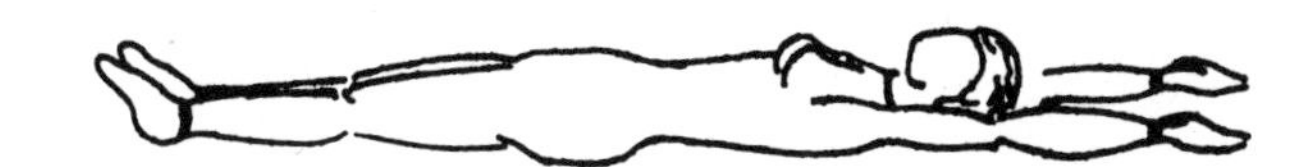

The Jackknife • Lie on your back with your arms stretched above your head and your legs straight out. *In one motion,* raise your legs off the floor (up to about a 60° angle) and raise your upper body until your fingers touch your toes. Your legs should be straight or almost-straight throughout, and your arms as close as possible to the same angle as your torso, so that your whole body folds sharply at the waist and balances on the top of your buttocks at the moment when fingers touch toes. Return to the prone position in one motion (coordination of upper and lower body is very important; one shouldn't get ahead of the other). The moment your hands and feet touch the floor, immediately repeat the movement. Repeat as many times as you can without overstraining. This exercise is much more difficult than the traditional sit-up. It benefits both the upper and lower abdominal muscles, and coordinates the two halves of the body around the energy of the waist region. Thirty-five continuous repetitions—without breaking form, wobbling, rolling, or changing rhythm—indicates excellent abdominal power and good coordination.

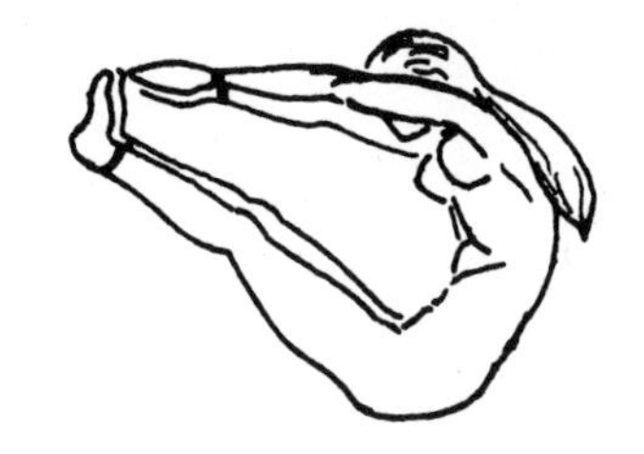

The Jackknife

The Back Raise • Lie on your stomach with your legs together and your arms spread-eagled on the floor, palms down. (One variation of this exercise is to keep your hands clasped behind your neck.) Have someone firmly hold down your feet and legs. Raise your arms, head, and chest as far as you can off the ground, then return to the prone position momentarily. Repeat as many times as you can without strain. This is a good one for spinal flexibility as well as strengthening all the muscles along the back, the shoulders, back of neck, buttocks, and backs of legs. Working on this exercise consists of increasing the number of repetitions you can perform without stopping *and* increasing the height to

The Back Raise

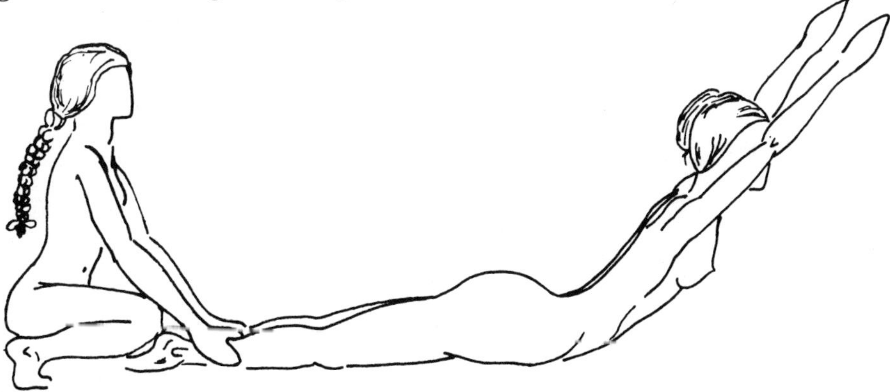

which you raise your head each time—that is, increasing the arch of your spine. Good back condition is indicated by 20 Back Raises to a height of about two feet, non-stop.

Sports

I'm not going to try to analyze the "health" value of every one of the dozens of sports that people play in America today. What I will do though, is to suggest some principles that may prove useful if you rely on sports as your major physical activity and outlet.

First: *Ambidextrous* (literally, "either-handed") sports are preferable to one-sided sports, because they develop balanced coordination and flow of energy rather than just benefiting the right- or left-hand side. For example, handball is preferable to tennis for this reason.

Second: *Continuous effort* is much better than interrupted or sporadic output because of its benefits to the heart and lungs (see Part Two, Chapter One) and for the greater total energy expenditure. Thus basketball is a healthier game than baseball.

Third: Sports in which the aim is *self-development,* rather than winning over another person or team, are more valuable to the player. Ultimately, winning and losing games against others is meaningless, beating somebody else in competition is pretty much pointless—but creating, developing, expressing, and enjoying *yourself* are involvements that last. For this reason, cross-country skiing or long-distance running are superior to competition golf or speedboat racing. If you see what I mean.

But there are no rules about these things. On the basis of your own character, your needs and desires, your strengths and weaknesses, you should make your own choices. It may well be that going down the block for a game of stickball with the guys is absolutely the best thing you could do at one particular time. Or it might be a long, solitary walk through the park, or the woods, that you need most. Or an hour of folk dancing, or an arm-wrestling contest, or anything. Who knows what you need better than you yourself?

Aerobics

Aerobic exercise has been defined and explained earlier in the book (Part II, Chapter One). There is an aerobic "system," though, devised by Major Kenneth Cooper of the USAF Medical Corps. After long, careful research and a great deal of practical experience, Cooper came up with a point system for the various kinds of aerobic exercise—such as running, cycling, and swimming. This point system is based on the amount of oxygen used up each minute per kilogram (2.2 pounds) of body weight by each particular exercise or activity.

According to this system, *30 points a week* is the *minimum* needed by persons of all ages and sexes to achieve the "training effect" (improved functioning of the heart, lungs, and other organs) and maintain an excellent state of health. Thirty points corresponds to running one mile six times a week, in 6½ to 8 minutes. Of course, there are many other ways to get the same 30 points—that is, to consume the same amount of oxygen per pound of body weight.

Keep in mind Dr. Cooper's 30-point weekly minimum; here are four of his point charts for aerobic exercises:

Walking 3 miles		*Running 1 mile*		*Swimming 400 yards*		*Cycling 4 miles*	
time	*points*	*time*	*points*	*time*	*points*	*time*	*points*
hour or longer	1½	20.00–14:30	1	13:20 plus	1	24 min plus	0
60:00–43:30	3	14:30–12:00	2	13:20–10:00	2½	24:00–16:00	2
43:30–36:00	6	12:00–10:00	3	10:00–6:40	3½	16:00–12:00	4
		10:00–8:00	4	under 6:40	5	under 12:00	6
		8:00–6:30	5				
		under 6:30	6				

KENNETH COOPER, M.D., *Aerobics*

Dr. Cooper advocates spreading your 30 (or more) points over at least three or four days—and preferably over six or seven days. He says to start slowly if you are out of condition, working up to that 30-plus level gradually. And, most important, he recommends keeping up your aerobic program, rain or shine, for your whole life. Since aerobic activity is most natural to the human animal, and most lacking in our sedentary, overcivilized lives—it's a very good idea!

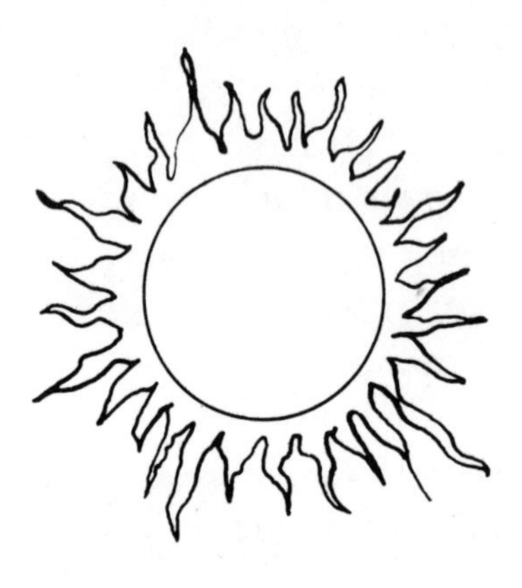

DIETARY SYSTEMS

Unfortunately, most dietary systems would like you to believe that if you just eat right (and there are some very different ideas about what "right" means) then everything else in your life will turn out well—you'll be free from disease, have plenty of energy, solve your emotional problems, and live long. I wish that were so, but it isn't. The most wholesome, nutritionally-balanced, and delicious meal won't do you much good if you're uptight when you eat it; or you're not really hungry but are substituting the food for affection or just for something to relieve your boredom; or you've been sitting on your behind for months, breathing poorly, and exerting almost no physical energy at all. There are many other factors that affect your health, besides the exact composition of your dietary intake. But food is *one* important factor, and warrants some attention. So here we go—all of the systems that follow contain at least some significant grain of truth about food and health, although I don't necessarily suggest buying the whole loaf.

Macrobiotics

Developed by Georges Ohsawa of Japan, this is a dietary-health system based on his version of the Yin-Yang principle. According to Ohsawa, certain foods—just like certain personality tendencies, physical events, and chemical elements—are Yin and certain ones are Yang. This is how he divides things up:

Yin	*Yang*
Female	Male
Vegetable	Animal
Cold	Heat
Silence	Sound
Dilation	Constriction
Lightness	Heaviness
Potassium	Sodium
Centrifugal movement	Centripetal movement

Health, Ohsawa says, is a balance of Yin and Yang—and is best achieved by balancing your food intake along those lines. Macrobiotics defines Yin foods as the sweet, soft, and sour, and those high in potassium—in the extreme, sugar, fruits, dairy products, yams, tomatoes, and eggplants (which are considered *too* Yin to eat at any time!). Yang foods are the bitter, salty, hard, and those rich in sodium; for example—carrots, garlic, wild game meat, hard apples, chestnuts, and ginseng are all very Yang foods. Of course, there is a gradation from very Yin through very Yang. The Macrobiotic ideal is to eat close to the middle and keep the Yin and Yang in the proper proportion.

Ohsawa figured that the single food most nearly perfect in terms of Yin-Yang balance for human beings (which meant to him a 5:1 proportion of potassium to sodium) was unpolished, organically-grown *brown rice.* This food became the central axis around which everything else was balanced—and was even proposed as a complete diet by itself, his famous Diet #7, which Ohsawa claimed could cure all manner of physical and mental disorders.

There have been many stories about Westerners, especially Americans, getting ill and even dying on strict Macrobiotic regimes. They may very likely be true. The point is that although Ohsawa's principles may appear sound, they don't take into account the fact that different people have very different internal chemical balances based on the variant factors of age, sex, race, genetic makeup, climate, type of work, physical condition, emotional state, and so on. Therefore they have very different food requirements. Certainly the dietary demands of a 40-year-old Caucasian housewife in the suburbs and the needs of a 20-year-old male Japanese farmworker are not likely to be exactly the same. If you'll excuse the pun, it seems clear that, at least in some cases, "one man's rice is another man's poison."

While the mono-diet for all people is a dangerous proposition, there is still a great deal of interesting information about food and health in Ohsawa's works that bears looking into. I myself don't follow anything remotely resembling the Macrobiotic diet, yet I can verify the tendencies of certain foods in terms of Yin and Yang qualities. For example, if I've just eaten a heavy Yang meal of meat with garlic, I feel better if I balance it off with some natural Yin sweet such as grapes or some other fruit. If I've just had a bowl of whole-grain cereal with milk and honey, which is pretty Yin, I like to eat a crisp, fresh, Yang-y apple afterwards. At least on this level, the Yin-Yang idea seems to correspond to my own *instincts* about eating, which are what I'm inclined to follow most of the time.

While Ohsawa's diet looks like a bad idea, especially in its extreme forms (the all-rice diet) if you want to stay alive, his heart was in the right place, and his criticism of the food-and-life style of modern man was quite apt. In the course of his research he devised this list of seven "levels of medicine," from the lowest and least developed to the highest, the ideal medicine:

a) "Symptomatic Medicine—Palliative treatment to remove symptoms." (This he said, and quite accurately, is mostly what we get today.)
b) "Prophylactic or Preventative Medicine." (A good doctor does this.)
c) "Art of Health—The study of the ways and means of acquiring physical health." (Highly recommended!)

d) "Macrobiotic Medicine—The art of rejuvenation and longevity." (A great idea, if we can find a way to *really* make it happen.)
e) "Sociomoral and Educational Medicine—Aims at the establishment of public health, freedom, and justice in society at large." (Right on, brother!)
f) "Philosophical Medicine—Directed to the mental plane of thought and judgment." (Pass the soy sauce.)
g) "Supreme Medicine—It is educational, biological, and physiological. Its aim is to make every man his own doctor, to permit the sick person to discover all by himself the cosmological conception of the universe as mirrored in his own body. It not only cures diseases of the present and future, but establishes a positive state of health and happiness."

G. OHSAWA, *You Are All Sanpaku*

Mucusless Diet

This system, developed by Dr. Arnold Ehret, defines all illnesses and all disorders as clogging of the body system with poisons of one kind or another—mucus being the internal matter that the unwanted toxic material resides in. The solution to almost every condition of ill health (he says) is to *fast* and allow your body to get rid of its poisons. When you are in good health you should eat *only fruits* (and fruit juices) *and green leafy vegetables*—which, according to Dr. Ehret, are the only foods that do not produce mucus.

This is an extremely low-protein diet that includes no meat, fish, or dairy products, no grains, and no legumes (beans); occasionally nuts are allowed. Inevitably, people following this diet lose a lot of weight, to the point where there is really very little "meat" left on their bones. The question of exact protein needs for maintaining life and health seems never to have been fully established—and, like most other factors, probably varies a great deal from person to person. (Things like climate, geography, exertion, age, and sex might affect one's protein requirements as well.)

Actually, protein is used primarily for tissue repair and body growth, and is only converted to energy for movement, body heat, and organ functioning when there is nothing else available. Mucusless theory holds that if you do not destroy your own body tissues through disease, intake of poisonous substances, or negative mental and emotional processes (like anxiety), then you hardly need any protein at all—and all your energy needs can be met by adequate amounts of fruit sugars.

The mucusless diet is called the "Garden of Eden" diet. It does not involve the killing of either plant or animal, but only the taking of Nature's fruits as they are provided for us. For this reason it is said to be the most spiritually "pure" diet. And it seems that this diet *does* correspond in its followers to the physical-mental-spiritual condition of closeness to nature, peacefulness, innocence, and clarity of mind—qualities we associate with life in the Garden. But, even if this is so, the diet may be very *inappropriate* for most of us, who don't live on untroubled tropical islands, but in a far more impure, violent, unholy, and unkind world, where to survive involves a struggle. We live in a world where to know Nature truly, as one of her children, makes you society's outcast, an opponent of the whole flow of our "civilization." We live in a world where to be free, and to love, do not come easily to us at all, but are victories to be won at some cost. This holiest of diets may not be enough for the lives most of us must lead.

An Eskimo shaman (a medicine man or holy man) once told the explorer Stefannson that the most difficult spiritual problem in the life of man is the fact that we must kill other things to go on living. My feeling about the mucusless diet is that it is no good as a permanent way of life in this most difficult of civilizations—but that, as a temporary cleansing and rejuvenating partial fast, to be followed for several days (or even up to several weeks), it is excellent. It really does help to rid your system of many troublesome wastes and toxic materials that have been clogging up your internal organs for years. And it may help cure any number of mental and physical disorders. If you try it, be sure to eat *only* unsprayed, untreated, organically-grown fruit and vegetables, and the fresh juices of these. Otherwise, if you're swallowing DDT, paraffin, mercury, and all the other things found in nonorganic foods, you're destroying the whole purpose of the diet—which is to *get rid of the poisons within your system.* Try the mucusless diet for a week and see how clean you feel!

Natural Organic Foods

This is a very loose "system" with one major principle: You should eat only natural foods (those that have not been processed, refined, or manufactured) that have been grown, or raised, *organically*—that is, without the use of any synthetic chemical fertilizers, sprays, treatments, or additives. Natural-organic foods is sort of the dietary wing of the ecology movement. It has become widespread in recent years as more and more people become aware of the incredible, criminal pollution and devitalization of most of our commercial, nonorganic foods. In its best form (though not the one most widely practiced), this diet is a joyous, relaxed acceptance of the earth's fruits (and meats and vegetables) just as Nature creates them. Organic foods *are* better for you, in every way: taste, looks, smell, texture, nutrition—and soul!

Did you know that there are literally *thousands* of pesticides, insecticides, bleaching agents, preservatives, coloring agents, artificial flavoring agents, desiccants, emulsifiers, stabilizers, texturizers, and other unnatural ingredients in your food and drink—almost all of them *poisons* when taken in sufficient quantity? Now although the sodium nitrite, say, in one hot dog is obviously not going to kill you, the built-up effect in your body, over the years, from ingesting those chemicals *will* undermine your health.

For example, if poisons are not excreted immediately, the liver—along with other internal organs—attempts to detoxify your system. Too much poison and the liver can be overstrained to the breaking point, leading to quite serious disorders such as toxic hepatitis. (Note: Hepatitis was a virtually unknown disease 100 years ago—when almost all foods were natural and organic.)

Too many poisonous substances in your system can also lead to serious deficiencies of the B and C vitamins, which are used up in the detoxification process. There's a huge array of illnesses and distressing symptoms that can result from this chronic low-level poisoning. A few of the more common examples are:

- Those decaying, discolored, corroded teeth may be due to too much sugar, lack of calcium and other essential minerals in your diet, improper care of teeth and gums; *or* they may be the result of the cumulative effects of any of the following commonly used commercial-food additives: nitrous oxide, bismuth, fluorides, tartaric acid, cadmium, chlorine, mercurials. Get the idea?
- Pale, anemic-looking skin might be caused by iron deficiency, some dire disease or blood ailment; *or* it might be due to eating commercial foods containing chlorine, lead arsenate, dinitrocresol, salicylates, vanadium pentoxide, or permanganate. You'd never know.
- Coughing and inflamed lungs may be the result of a cold, bronchitis, emphysema, pneumonia; *or* the result of ferrous chloride, hydrochloric acid, pyridine, zinc oxide, formaldehyde, sulfur dioxide, chloropicrin, sulfur chloride, chlorosulfonic acid, or any of a number of chemical additives in *your* food!
- That pounding headache might not just be caused by tension; it could be due to methyl bromide, 2-aminopyrine, caffeine, carbon disulfide, lead, chlorine, nicotine, parathion, or phenylhydrazine.

- Feeling fatigued, worn out for no reason? Could be anemia, mononucleosis, malnutrition, or some other disease; but then again, it could be something you bought at the supermarket last month, one of those brightly packaged numbers containing salicylate, strychnine, parathion, lead, bromides, mercury compounds, pyridine, nicotine, methyl chloride, methyl bromide, carbon disulfide, zinc chloride, diethylstilbestrol.

This list goes on and on, but I'll stop here. (I assume you get the message.) But even more deadly than the presence of all these poisonous ingredients in our foods is the *absence* of essential natural nutrients, lost by modern agricultural methods and processing. This is how it happens:

Imagine an organic tomato garden. Let's say that every 15-foot row of this naturally fertilized, composted, unsprayed garden produces, on the average, 50 pounds of tomatoes. Let's also assume, for the sake of argument, that there are 100 milligrams of naturally-occurring iron in the soil of every 15-foot row, which is available to be absorbed into the tomatoes growing there. (Iron is one of the essential macronutrients vital to human health.) So we get 50 pounds of harvested tomatoes, with 100 milligrams of iron—that is, 2 milligrams of iron in every one-pound tomato.

Now imagine a 15-foot section of tomato plants on a huge modern commercial farm. First of all, the soil has not been enriched by composting and organic fertilizing, so it has fewer available minerals than the organic garden soil. (Iron-deficient soil *has* in fact been reported in most of the 50 states, especially the East coast from Florida to Massachusetts, certain areas of the Southwest, and California's Imperial Valley—the greatest fruit-growing area in America.) Let's say the 15-foot row therefore has only 50 milligrams of available iron in the soil.

The soil and the plants themselves have been treated with various chemicals to make them produce larger

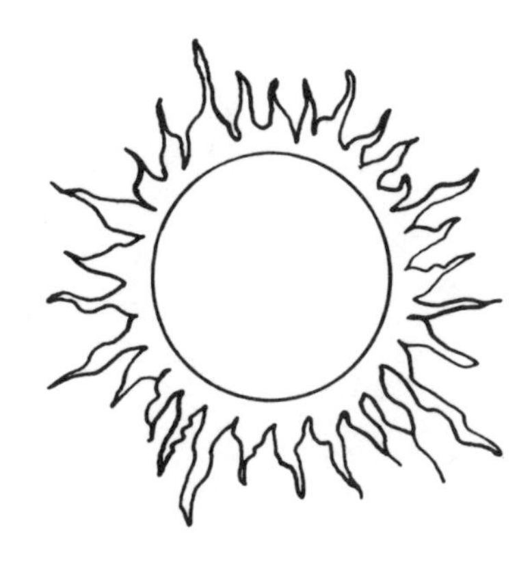

fruit—and more of them on each single plant, occupying the same area of soil as an organic plant. So *100* pounds of tomatoes are produced in the 15-foot row. This is called "progress." But the amount of nutrients available from the soil has not increased—it is, as we said, 50 milligrams. Thus 100 pounds of tomatoes are grown, with 50 milligrams of iron in them—that is, one-half milligram in every one-pound tomato. This is one-quarter as much iron as there was in the organically-grown tomato!

While these are all made-up figures, used to illustrate the point, the real situation is just like this—and not just for tomatoes but for all fruits and vegetables and grains and even meats! (The domestic animals are given non-organically grown feed, and are often injected with various growth hormones to fatten them up.) And it's true not only for iron but for every one of the essential vitamins, minerals, and other nutrients that you depend on your food to provide. Every day you are paying for and eating "empty food" that looks good, probably weighs a lot—but contains only a small fraction of its natural nutritional value!

Take commercial white bread, for example. First of all, it's chock-full of many lovely little chemicals: mercury that the seeds were treated with; pesticides that were sprayed onto the growing wheat; chlorine dioxide that was used to bleach the flour (a dangerous explosive poison, by the way); ammonium chloride that was put in as a dough conditioner; polyoxyethylene, a softener; ditertiary-butyl-paraCresol, an antioxidant; butter yellow dye, a coal-tar derivative used to suggest that the bread actually has butter or egg yolk in it (just like mother used to make!); and finally, calcium propionate (usually the only one of these that will actually be listed on the package), a mold inhibitor so that your bread, already permanently softened, can stay "fresh" on the shelf (even for weeks). But not only are all these delicious ingredients going into your daily bread (and there are a lot more not mentioned here)—the two most vital, nutritionally rich parts of the wheat itself, the bran and the germ, have been totally removed! This is by far the greatest crime of all regarding bread.

Before 1910, heart disease was virtually unknown in the United States. In that year they started removing the bran from wheat. And later, the germ—which is rich in B vitamins and is also one of nature's greatest sources of vitamin E, a nutrient essential to good heart condition and physical endurance.

In short, commercial white bread is full of harmful additives *and* almost worthless nutritionally. The natural-organic alternative is to buy *whole-grain* bread made with untreated flour and no chemicals. Or, better yet, bake your own! The result is a much tastier and infinitely healthier food: *real* bread.

The principles of natural-organic eating are sound and I do endorse them. But the tendency to become fanatically *anxious* about what you eat (or about what other people are eating) should be studiously avoided. At one time I was so crazy about natural diet that I wouldn't lick a postage stamp for fear of "contaminating" myself with the poisonous glue! That's what I mean by fanaticism, folks, and I hope you pass it by.

As Zorba the Greek and I said earlier, your body is a remarkable machine that can take what it needs from almost any kind of food and get rid of the rest—providing that you maintain good health with plenty of exercise, *and* a healthy relaxed outlook on life. If you're worrying about what you eat all the time, that can make you sicker than anything! Just pay attention in an easy, happy way, try to avoid the heavily treated and highly synthetic foods, and gradually steer your eating pattern back to the natural. After a while, a Coke or a maraschino cherry or a piece of white bread won't even look like food to you.

Vitamins and Other Pills

The theory behind vitamin pills and other dietary supplements is simple: Your nutritional needs (so the pill advocates claim) can't be met by your diet alone. Because of the low nutritional content of most available foods, they say, and the added stresses of modern living, plus the detoxification requirements from our polluted food, air, and water, certain vitamins, minerals, and proteins have to be added.

A very strong case can be made for vitamin C, which is used up when your system gets rid of poisons or is under any kind of stress—either external or internal. Cigarette smoking, booze, grass, LSD, fear, anxiety, pain, nervousness, physical ailments of all kinds—from colds to broken bones—seem to deplete your body's store of C. Therefore your body demands that you get more. Linus Pauling, the Nobel prize-winning scientist, regards vitamin C as essential, in huge doses, to prevent colds and resist all the infectious diseases common in overpopulated society, and to maintain your internal health amidst the stresses of life today. He himself takes 6 *grams* of vitamin C per day, which is equivalent to twenty-four 250-milligram pills, the commonest size C supplement. This may or may not be extremism—you'll have to figure it out for yourself.

The vitamin pill industry is big business these days, so you certainly can't trust what *they* say; they'd have you believe that you need to be popping 10 or 12 different pills at every meal just to stay alive. Obviously, man in a more natural state (like the Indians before the arrival of the white man, who in general enjoyed superb health and suffered few if any of the diseases now filling our hospitals and cemeteries) didn't need vitamin pills. And it's clear that the more natural and wholesome your diet is today, the less likely you are to need supplements of any kind.

The catch is that air pollution, impure water supplies, cigarette smoke, and a hundred other unavoidable toxins *do* change your dietary needs—especially for C. And unless your food is grown or raised on rich, organically-fertilized soil, it is probably deficient in at least several of the most essential macronutrients (iron, calcium, phosphorous, potassium) and vital trace minerals (magnesium, copper, iodine, manganese, cobalt, zinc, and others). So what do you do?

You can drive yourself crazy trying to figure out exactly which of these nutrients your diet lacks, exactly how much you need of it, and what foods or pills to get it from—the Adelle Davis books are probably the most reasonable example of this approach. If you are in very bad health right now, or seem generally prone to illness, injury, or emotional problems, you might do well to take up this kind of personal research. Your diet may really be lacking some essential nutrients—and that lack may be the direct cause, on a physical level at least, for the disorder. Whether or not changing your diet will solve the *whole* problem—even if the immediate symptoms disappear—is debatable.

For example, there have been a lot of reports in the press recently about curing schizophrenia and other mental-emotional disorders with megavitamin therapy. That is, the patient is given very large dosages of certain vitamins (B vitamins, in the case of schizophrenia) and reportedly achieves an astonishing recovery. Well, it's not yet clear whether these "successes" are what they're claimed to be. But even if the reports are correct, does that mean that schizophrenia, or any other psychotic disorder, is just a vitamin deficiency? I don't think so. Certainly every mental or emotional condition is also a chemical and electrical pattern in your body, so that rebalancing a chemical deficiency (lack of thiamine, for example) with vitamin therapy may *temporarily* alleviate the condition. But the underlying problem in the person's whole mindbody system that *created* the illness pattern has not yet been dealt with. So the disease will probably reappear, although not necessarily in the same form. Human beings are complicated life-systems, not machines to be fueled and oiled and started up. Unless the *whole* person is treated, no cure can be really successful.

The question of vitamin and mineral supplements is still open. You probably do need more C than you are getting in your daily diet, unless you eat huge quantities of citrus fruits and other foods rich in C; and you could probably use some vitamin E for better heart condition —especially if you eat a lot of white breads and commercial baked goods (as opposed to whole-grain foods). On the other hand, the best remedy is to return to your senses and instincts about food, body chemistry, nutrition—through plenty of natural movement, deep breathing, relaxation, emotional liberation—and let your body inform you of its requirements! This is better than a hundred nutrition books and a truckload of pills.

Fasting

This is the oldest method in the world for restoring health and vitality. It is mentioned in the Bible and in other sources thousands of years old. Animals also fast when they are not well—fasting is one of Nature's great cures!

The principle of fasting is simple: Cleanse and purify yourself internally; deny nourishment to bacteria that are making you ill; rid yourself of all the waste products clogging your circulatory, digestive, respiratory, and glandular systems—and your health will be restored.

Total fasting means to eat no solid food and to drink only pure water. (Sometimes lemon juice and honey, or other fruit juices, can be added to the water, but in small amounts.) There are also modified or *partial* fasts, such as the Mucusless fast (only fresh fruits and green, starchless vegetables); the Macrobiotic fast (boiled brown rice only); the raw-juice fast (several glasses of *fresh* fruit and vegetable juices every day); and any mono-diet (only *one* food is eaten, and in small quantities).

Fasting not only cleanses your body but brings deep psychological and spiritual changes as well. Many great religious leaders are said to have fasted before their enlightenment: Jesus went 40 days in the wilderness; Buddha fasted sitting beneath the Bodhi tree; American Plains Indians fasted and took sweat baths (another cleansing method) before going into the wilderness on solitary "vision quests."

Our daily lives are built around meals. Eating reflects our culture, personality, life-style, habits, and fixed ideas. Often we don't know what we're eating, why we're eating it, or if it's any good for us—but we eat. Fasting takes you out of the breakfast-lunch-dinner cycle, breaks the old unhealthy patterns, brings you to a larger perspective. Fasting can not only change your dietary habits and your outlook on food, it can also expand your awareness of yourself and others. Fasting lets you see behind the surface appearances of things, to the deeper forces that really shape the world—it puts you in touch with a "greater reality." And, as a relaxed exercise in self-discipline, it teaches you that your life—even in its most fundamental functions—can be made more conscious, altered, and improved.

Before telling you how to start a short fast, one note of warning. Some of the toxic substances you take in are neither excreted immediately *nor* detoxified by the liver or other organs. Instead they are stored in your body semi-permanently. DDT, for example, which we get a lot of because most crops are sprayed with it at one time or another (including feed grains, which are then fed to animals whose meat and/or milk will contain DDT): DDT is *stored* in the fatty tissues of your body. When you fast, or go on a crash reducing diet, the fat begins to get used up for energy in the absence of your daily intake. As the fat "melts," the DDT stored there gets released into your bloodstream in quite concentrated form—and can actually poison you! There have been several reports in the past few years of deaths from this kind of internal DDT poisoning, mainly among very fat people who went on extreme reducing diets. Needless to say, DDT is only one of many poisons in your body that may start "moving" when you start fasting. So, before undertaking any fasting at all, you should taper off by eating less than normal for several days at least, and eat as many natural foods as possible. Your first couple of fasts should be no longer than a day or two, to avoid the danger of too much toxic material being passed out of you at one time. Also, you should keep exercising during this period, both for the stimulation it gives your circulatory system and for *sweating*—one of your body's great mechanisms for getting rid of poisons. (Steam baths and saunas are also good for this purpose.)

In this beginning, trial period of tapering off and one-day fasts, you should stop at any signs of serious discomfort or malfunction and start eating normally again. Fasting is one of the most valuable health techniques—but it must be undertaken with great care, especially at the outset.

Assuming you have already de-poisoned yourself a little with a tapering-off diet, more natural foods and less chemicals, a lot of good sweaty exercise, and a few short (one-day) fasts, you're ready to start fasting for real. The first days are the hardest, both because of your *appetite,* which is making you crave something to eat even though you don't really need it, and because the long-accumulated poisons inside you are starting to pass out, and that passage never feels too good.

Your first serious fast should be somewhere between three and seven days, but no longer. Drink plenty of pure water—at least five glasses every day. Water helps wash out the impurities, especially those that are going to pass through your kidneys. And keep active in a light, relaxed, and easy fashion—after a while you'll begin to feel pretty energetic! Sweating, relaxation, and plenty of sleep are essential to proper fasting. Tension and stress will only inject more unpleasant chemicals (this time internally produced) into your bloodstream, hindering your digestive organs in their cleansing process. So take it easy.

Fasting is a meditation with respect to food. It is a journey *inside* your everyday reality—and it may change your life. Try it and see.

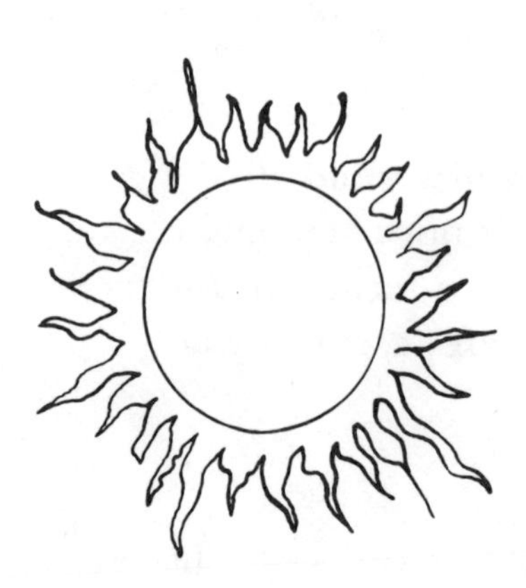

SEXUAL HEALTH SYSTEMS

Mental illness is a disturbance in the natural capacity for love. In the case of orgastic impotence, from which a vast majority of humans are suffering, biological energy is dammed up, thus becoming the source of all kinds of irrational behavior. . . . The vital energies, under natural conditions, regulate themselves spontaneously, without compulsive duty or compulsive morality. . . .

The character structure of man today . . . is characterized by an *armoring against nature within himself and against social misery outside himself.* This armoring of the character is the basis of loneliness, helplessness, craving for authority, fear of responsibility, mystical longing, sexual misery, of impotent rebelliousness as well as of resignation of an unnatural and pathological type. . . .

Owing to the split in the human character structure of today, nature and culture, instinct and morality, sexuality and achievement, are considered incompatible. That *unity of culture and nature, work and love, morality and sexuality* for which mankind is forever longing, this unity will remain a dream so long as man does not permit the satisfaction of the biological demands of natural (orgastic) sexual gratification. . . .

Orgastic potency is the capacity for surrender to the flow of biological energy without any inhibition, the capacity for *complete discharge of all dammed-up sexual excitation* through *involuntary pleasurable contractions of the body.* . . .

[The] fundamental principle is the restoration of bio-psychic motility by means of dissolving rigidities ("armorings") of the character and the musculature.

WILHELM REICH, *The Function of the Orgasm*

Reich's life work was based upon sexual energy. He held that true mental and emotional health is always rooted in the bodily experience. No one is healthy, he said, unless their sex life is completely fulfilling—which means, not just "well-performed" but totally instinctual and unconscious at the point of climax. He developed several interconnected methods of treating mental-physical-emotional disorders, including a kind of psychotherapy; certain types of deep muscle massage; exercises for loosening up areas of rigidity and tension; and the "orgone box," a device to accumulate *orgone* energy (sex or life-energy, similar to ki or prana) in a person whose flow was blocked. Probably his most important contribution was the discovery that neuroses, psychoses, and in fact all personality characteristics are not confined to the mind but are also *located in the body* as specific patterns of tension, rigidity, looseness, painfulness, sensitivity or desensitivity, free flow of biological energy (life-energy) or its obstruction. This discovery allowed many emotional, sexual, and mental disorders to be treated more directly through the body—instead of through years of orthodox psychoanalysis.

Today there are in private practice a small number of Reichian therapists who use some of the methods just described; there are also a larger number of therapists using related methods whose principles derive from Reich's discoveries.

One of the best known of these is Alexander Lowen, a former student of Reich. His system is called Bioenergetics. Lowen deals with people on both the psychic and physical levels, but emphasizes bodily functioning as the basis for emotional, sexual, and mental health. He believes the two most important life-functions are *breathing* and *movement.* (He points out that death is indicated by stopped breathing, total lack of movement —and loss of feeling. Despite this, many people go on "living" with shallow, constricted breathing patterns, awkward and limited mobility, and very little in the way of feeling, either.)

Lowen defines health not just as the absence of disease, illness, or pain—but positively, as a balanced state of beauty, grace, pleasure, and unobstructed flow of life-energy. His Reichian principles are important ones, so I'll let him speak for himself:

> In a healthy individual thinking and feeling follow parallel lines, reflecting the unity of the personality. In a neurotic individual thinking often opposes feeling. . . . The moment one has to think about moving, the spontaneous flow of feeling through the body is interrupted. The break in rhythmic movement produces a condition of gracelessness. All animals are graceful in their movements. . . . Primitive people retain much of their animal grace, which is progressively lost in the civilizing process. It is lost when a person is not free to follow his instincts and feelings. . . . The person endowed with grace . . . is open because no tensions restrict the flow of feeling. . . . He is warm because his energy is not bound in emotional conflicts. He has more energy and therefore more feeling. He gives pleasure to others without effort, for every movement of his body is a source of pleasure to himself and others. In a human being the lack of physical grace is due to chronic muscular tensions that block the involuntary physical movements of the body. Each tension pattern represents an emotional conflict that was resolved by the inhibition of certain impulses. . . .
>
> The true test of gracefulness is in the normal everyday movements of life: walking, talking, cooking a meal, or playing with a child. Beauty of bodily form and grace of bodily movement are the outer or objective manifestations of health. Pleasure is the inner or subjective experience of health. Health is indivisible.
>
> ALEXANDER LOWEN, *Pleasure*

Here is a simple body position used in Bioenergetic therapy to restore feeling to the legs and feet: Stand with your feet slightly apart and toes turned a little inward, knees slightly bent. Bend over as if you were touching your toes—but don't put any weight onto your hands. Keep the balance in your feet, allowing your upper body to hang totally relaxed and loose (*including* your head, shoulders, and neck). Breathe easily and freely, with your mouth open. Lowen says that your legs should vibrate or tremble after you've been in this position a little while, but that this is normal: "All alive bodies vibrate in stress conditions."

Reich's discoveries—which covered a broad range of subjects from psychology and social theory to biology, education, and cosmology—contain the scientific basis for the transformation from the modern, overcivilized, imbalanced, repressed, amoral character to new Whole Person who is sexually, emotionally, physically, mentally, and socially healthy. Reich's work is of tremendous significance in the further development of man on this planet. Here are just a few of Reich's discoveries:

1. Sexual health is the precondition for the total health of every human being—man, woman, or child. Sexual health means *self*-regulation of erotic drives (that is, freedom from repression, guilt, anxiety, and other pressures) and complete surrender in orgasm.
2. Inhibited or repressed natural energies turn into "negative" forces such as hate, sadism, dependency, helplessness, etc.
3. With respect to the diagnosis and treatment of all sexual, emotional, characterological disorders, the "mind" and the "body" are inseparable and interconnected.
4. Our society (like almost all patriarchal, authoritarian, sexually unliberated, hierarchic societies) cruelly stifles the natural feelings of love, sexuality, movement, and responsibility—in almost all people. In their place are substituted obedience, competition, desire for wealth and power, social amorality. This process takes its most virulent form in the education

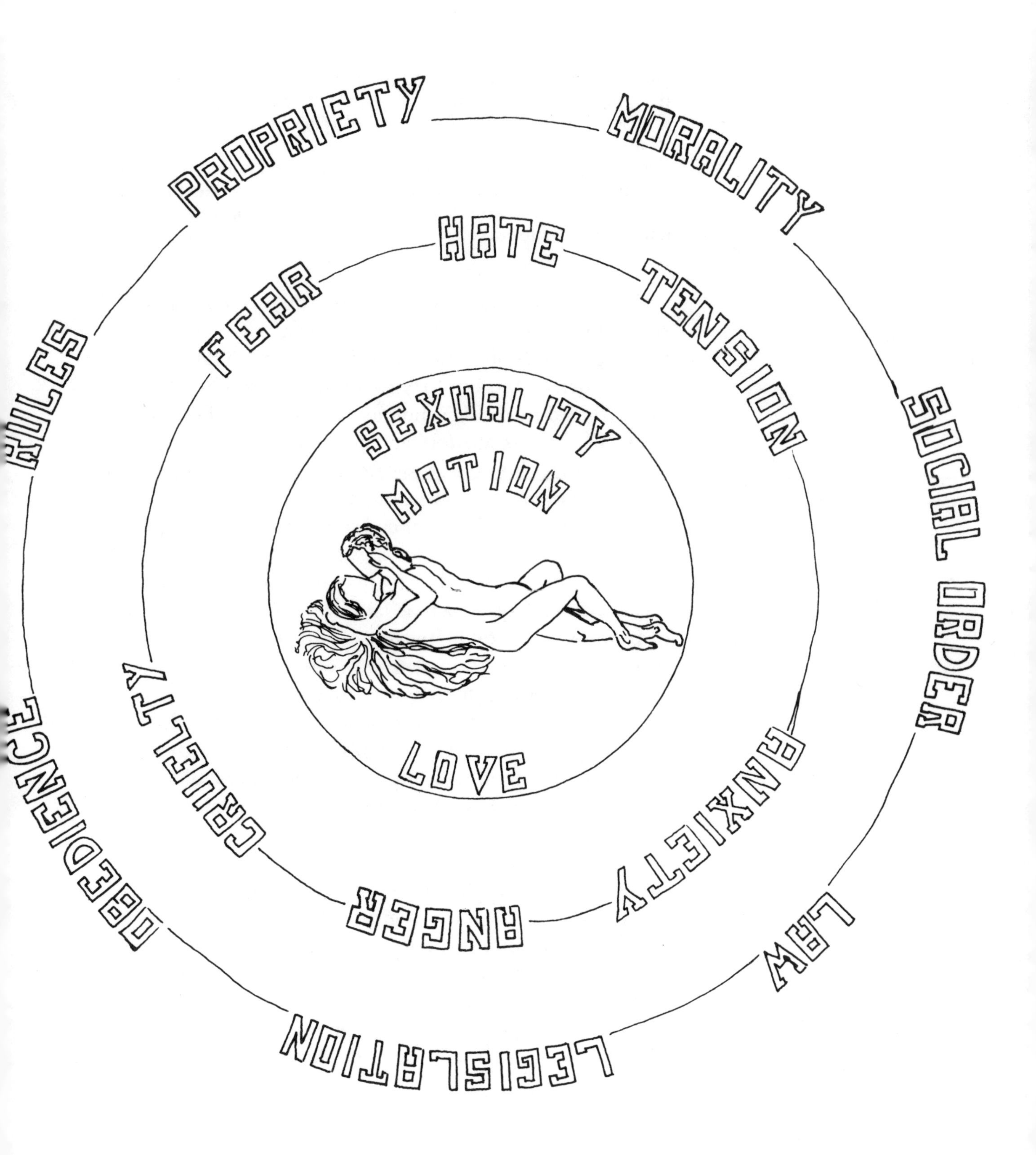
PROPRIETY
MORALITY
SOCIAL ORDER
LAW
LEGISLATION
OBEDIENCE
RULES
HATE
TENSION
ANXIETY
ANGER
CRUELTY
FEAR
SEXUALITY
MOTION
LOVE

and rearing of children through adolescence. Reich believed that only a non-repressive yet responsible upbringing of children could produce a generation of truly healthy men and women.

5. *Orgone,* or sexual energy, is present (and verifiable, measurable) in all healthy living things—and in fact is found throughout the earth, the atmosphere, and the entire universe as a kind of basic life-force.

Reich's work has produced and influenced a whole spectrum of new sexual and psychosomatic therapies, ranging from Bioenergetics and Sensitivity Training and Deep-Muscle Massage to Structural Integration (Rolfing), "Third-force" Psychology, and Primal Therapy. Even the famous Masters and Johnson sex clinics have been strongly influenced by Reich's ideas. The basis for the tremendous success in curing sexual disorders—which is the basis for all these systems' successes—is the *breaking down of all blocks to the natural flow of sexual and emotional energy.* These blocks may exist as attitudes, ideas, and feelings (such as lack of confidence, feelings of powerlessness or helplessness, anxiety of any kind, fear of letting go, fear of losing control, repression of anger or of love). Or they may exist in the form of physical dysfunctions and imbalances (such as reduced breathing, muscle tensions, suppressed pain, body weakness or clumsiness). But ultimately the "mental" and "physical" problems must be seen as interconnected, and must both be dealt with.

The Masters and Johnson clinics, for example, work on both levels simultaneously. On the one hand, through intensive psychological counseling of the individuals and couples under treatment—with respect to their attitudes, feelings, anxieties, character tendencies, and relationships, plus a careful, systematic establishment of a nonthreatening, reinforcing, relaxed, and pleasurable context in which the physical reordering can take place. On the other hand, the clinics work through actual sex "training" to cure impotence, frigidity, premature ejaculation, and other such common yet quite serious sexual problems. These methods have been described quite well in a number of available books. The point to remember, though, is that the psychological and the physical therapies *together* form the complete "cure"; either one alone is not enough.

The Reichian systems and those influenced by Reich afford the clearest available paths out of the sexual-emotional disaster area of our culture. I recommend a study of Reich's principles and methods to everyone who feels the need for such a "way out."

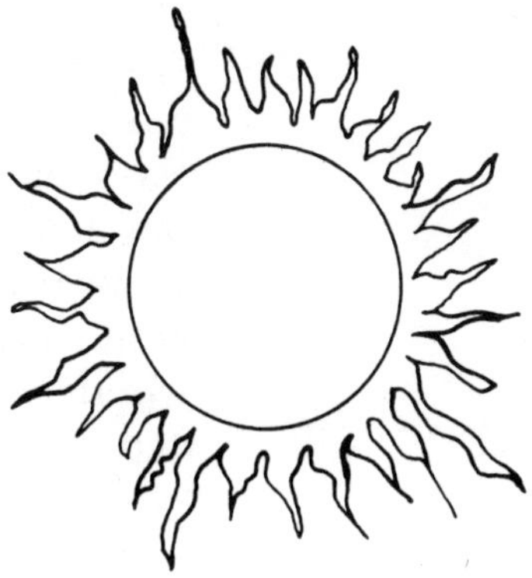

THE BATES EYE SYSTEM

Vision can be improved; the secret is relaxation of the mind and eye.

MARGARET DARST CORBETT

In the process of seeing, mind, eyes and nervous system are intimately associated to form a single whole. Anything which affects one element in this whole exercises an influence upon the other elements.

ALDOUS HUXLEY

In the course of time I discovered that myopia and hypermetropia, like astigmatism, could be produced at will; that myopia was not, as we have so long believed, associated with the use of the eyes at the near-point, but with a strain to see distant objects, strain at the near-point being associated with hypermetropia; that no error of refraction was ever a constant condition; and that the lower degrees of refractive error could be eliminated, while higher degrees could be improved. . . . In making these statements I am well aware that I am controverting the practically undisputed teaching of ophthalmological science for the better part of a century, but I have been driven to my conclusions by the facts, and so slowly that I am now surprised at my own hesitation. . . . The object of all the methods used in the treatment of imperfect sight without glasses is to secure rest or relaxation, first of the mind and then of the eyes. Rest always improves the vision. Effort always lowers it. Persons who wish to improve their visions should begin by proving these facts to themselves.

DR. WILLIAM H. BATES

This is a unique system for restoring natural vision without the use of glasses. But Bates' approach to the whole problem is so beautiful and so healthy that I want to include it as a perfect example of the integrated bodymind approach. Also, since millions of people now wear glasses and continue to suffer from eye problems of one kind or another, it's an appropriate subject to bring up.

Bates was a trained and practicing ophthalmologist, and discovered most of the principles of his system in the course of his objective, unprejudiced scientific research. He made thousands of observations with the retinoscope—a device that enabled him to look into the retina of the human eye while that eye was looking at things.

His final theory was simple, and revolutionary: Almost all eyesight disorders are the result of *strain* (that is, either mental or physical tension). The eye in a natural, relaxed state sees perfectly. But any difficulty, from the pain of stepping on a tack to the stress of entering a roomful of unfamiliar people, or the pressure of a competitive school classroom, can produce tensions in the muscles around the eye—which cause "errors of refraction," or imperfect vision. People who have bad eyesight for many years actually have chronic tensions that reduce their eyes' functioning.

Glasses, says Bates, are artificial crutches and only make you dependent on them—which is why people with glasses frequently have to get stronger and stronger lenses. At their best, glasses never cure your poor vision, but allow you to see reasonably well despite the chronic tension of your eyes-and-mind.

Instead of glasses, Bates suggests several different methods by which people can attain normal, or even better-than-normal, natural eyesight. He gives more than one way to go about healing your eyes, because to keep trying and straining away at a method which is not working for you will only create more tension and will defeat the whole system's purpose. The essence of good seeing is *relaxation:*

> The remedy is not to avoid either near work or distant vision, but to get rid of the mental strain which underlies the imperfect functioning of the eye at both points. It has been demonstrated in thousands of cases that this can be done. . . .
>
> To secure permanent relaxation sometimes requires considerable time and much ingenuity. The same method cannot be used with everyone. The ways in which people strain to see are infinite, and the methods used to relieve the strain must be almost equally varied. Whatever the method that brings most relief, however, the end is always the same, namely, relaxation. By constant repetition and frequent demonstration and by all means possible, the fact must be stressed that perfect sight can be obtained *only* by relaxation. . . .
>
> Temporary conditions may contribute to the strain to see which results in the production of errors of refraction, but its foundation lies in wrong habits of thought. . . .
>
> It is as natural for the eye to see as it is for the mind to acquire knowledge, and any effort in either case not only is useless but defeats the end in view. . . . The eye with normal sight never *tries* to see. . . . Whenever the eye tries to see, it at once ceases to have normal vision. . . . The act of seeing is passive.
>
> WILLIAM BATES, M.D., *Better Eyesight Without Glasses*

The relaxation required for normal vision is the type that Huxley calls "dynamic relaxation"—that is, maintaining an ease of the mind, nerves, and muscles while working, moving, and functioning. Dynamic relaxation is the secret of all skill—and of perfect vision. Here are several of the Bates practices for promoting it:

The Elephant Swing

Large muscular activity, particularly rhythmic motion, soothes the nerves. ("Immobility and rigidity are the products of civilization and the beginning of tension and nerves. So, free the large muscles of their tension first by rhythmic motion. These large voluntary muscles will transfer sympathetically their vibrations to the more minute involuntary muscles, including those of the eyes which start unconsciously their many shifts per second necessary for normal vision."—Margaret Darst Corbett, *Help Yourself to Better Sight*)

Stand with your feet comfortably apart and sway slowly from one foot to the other. Turn in the direction of your weight change, allowing hips, shoulders, head, and eyes to swing easily together in one direction, then the other. You can turn up on the toes of the rear foot each time. Keep your eyes open and relaxed—make no attempt to *see* anything, just let the world go by. Breathe in and out as you turn, in coordination with your swing. (Counting your swings out loud is helpful.) The maintenance of deep, relaxed, natural breathing is essential to normal vision. (Breath-holding, on the other hand, is a common manifestation of bodymind tension.) Be sure all your muscles are relaxed and loose, and that you are swinging easily, gracefully, and pleasurably. Do this *at least* 100 times, morning and evening, and it will benefit both your state of mind and your vision.

The Metal Disk

> (With your eyes closed) "1. Imagine that in your hand you hold a heavy metal disk the size and weight of a silver dollar. It has a smooth hole

through the center. Thread the disk on a white cord about a foot long. Pick up one end of the cord between the thumb and finger of the left hand, and the other end between thumb and finger of the right hand. Hold the cord taut to make a white line, disk in the center, at a comfortable distance before your face. Now point your nose at the fingers of one hand, then slide your mental vision across the white cord to the other hand, slowly, rhythmically, back and forth. The metal disk in the center seems to shift a little from one side to the other, in the opposite direction.

2. Now allow the cord to loosen a bit so that the heavy disk hangs low in the middle. Start the disk swinging gently toward you and away from you as you would rock a hammock, rhythmically back and forth, back and forth, not too fast.

3. Now let the hammock-swing gain momentum, higher and higher, until you take it all the way around like a jump rope, mentally remembering the disk as it completes its circle around and around.

4. Now 'let the old cat die,' as children say, and the disk again rocks gently to and from you like a hammock. It is fun to do the jump-rope swing around the opposite way, then again swing the hammock gently, to and fro.

5. Finally, and without a jerk, tighten the cord until it again forms a taut white line before your face, the disk in the center. Slide your mental vision across the cord from one hand slowly to the other. Once more, the disk will move with rhythm from one side to the other.

If you have done this with interest and ease, when the eyes are opened they will feel easy and loose and the vision will be improved."

MARGARET DARST CORBETT, *Help Yourself to Better Sight*

Myopia (nearsightedness)

The oblique muscles, which encircle the eye, and whose action makes the eyeball longer (that is, focused for near-vision), are chronically tightened in the nearsighted person. This tension may be due to any fear or anxiety or straining to see a distant object—or just to unhealthy seeing habits of the bodymind. Some of the Bates practices for cure of myopia are:

1. Pay attention to *shape*. Analyze things (with glasses off) as to their size, height, width, contours, edges, form. Even if the object appears blurry, the mind can use the shape information in interpreting (that is, "seeing") the object.
2. Practice shifting all over an object rather than staring at it without moving your eyes. The healthy eye is in continuous and very rapid motion; the unhealthy eye stares, strains, and does not move. Go over things you see for all their details, moving constantly from point to point. But stay relaxed.
3. Become interested (again, with glasses *off*) in things at a distance—in fact, become interested in distance itself. Most nearsighted people are afraid of distance and narrow their "world-view" accordingly. Look out as far as you can!
4. Go to the movies and watch without your glasses. The continuously moving images make staring impossible; your eyes have to shift, and this is good for them. Sit up close to start with; as your vision improves (over a period of days, weeks, or months), move further and further back.
5. Never allow your eyes to get tired. Periodically rest them (by closing them and by palming—which will be described shortly). Be sure to breathe deeply, and often. And never, never *try* to see something; just relax and let yourself see.

Glasses

Glasses are miserable devices. They lower your perception of color and form, contract your field of vision, make objects appear smaller (the convex lens) or larger (the concave lens) than they really are. You must produce the kind and degree of refractive error the glasses were made to correct if you are to see clearly through them—even when your actual vision might be better than that. And, worst of all, you get to rely on them, like crutches, weakening whatever visual health you do have, requiring stronger and stronger lenses, and allowing your natural seeing habits to deteriorate.

The Bates system holds that you should get rid of your glasses—but it is best to do so gradually, as your vision improves. Don't try to drive your car, for example, or do some other dangerous work without your glasses, when your vision is still imperfect. Don't strain and force yourself to see things without your glasses—this defeats the whole purpose of the system. Instead, go without them whenever you *feel* you can do so comfortably, securely, beneficially:

> There are many places and conditions where there is no mental pressure and a nearsighted eye can safely use its own power, as, for example, dressing in the morning, eating breakfast, riding as a passenger, etc. This builds visual acuity. Be on the alert for all these opportunities. The eye loves its freedom.
>
> MARGARET DARST CORBETT, *Help Yourself to Better Sight*

Presbyopia (hypermetropia, or farsightedness)

Everyone believes that farsightedness is an inevitable product of getting old. Bates and his followers say that it is caused by tension and other negative mind-eye-body patterns. Here are several Bates recommendations for farsighted people:

1. Breathe deeply and frequently, especially when you are looking at things up close and reading.
2. Blink frequently to rest your eyes and lubricate them.
3. Take sun or strong light on your closed eyelids (and even on the noncentral portions of the open eye for short flashes), and practice palming and closing your eyes frequently.
4. Keep your eyeballs feeling soft at all times—by loosening the lids, relaxing facial muscles, reducing eyebrow pressure. Check your eyes for softness often, and restore the feeling when you lose it.
5. Avoid staring. Avoid tension. Never *try* to read print. Use good light always. Read rapidly to avoid the stare habit. Prac-

tice looking at small, familiar things in a relaxed and gradually closer way. Never strain to see!

The Bates system includes many other methods—such as Centralization, Blinking and Flashing, use of Memory and Imagination, Sunning, Relaxing the Five Senses, and others—for the purpose of restoring natural vision without glasses. Several excellent books are available describing the system (see page 209), and there are trained instructors all around the world teaching natural vision. There is just one more practice from the Bates system I want to tell you about—for relaxing your eyes and reducing the strain that undermines perfect sight. It's called *Palming:*

Sit or lie down in a comfortable position, and relax. Close your eyes and cover them with your cupped palms so that your fingers cross on your forehead. Rest your eyes; rest your mind. If you see only perfect black (that is, absolute darkness) then you are relaxed and your eyes—at least while you're palming—are functioning normally.

The degree to which you do *not* see perfect black, but instead see spots, colors, shapes, or anything else, is an index of how much you are still straining, still tense, still suffering from wrong habits of thought—and therefore still seeing imperfectly.

Use your imagination, your memory, and plenty of time to help you see only perfect black when palming. (For example, remember the way something looks that is absolutely jet-black.) The practice of palming rests your eyes and also reacquaints them with the natural, effortless pattern of good seeing. Sleeping does not do this—in fact it has been shown that your eyes often strain as much (or more) when you're asleep as when you're awake. Palming is a meditation for your eyes. To be successful, it must be based upon relaxing your mind as well. Palming can't be overdone, and I recommend it

Palming

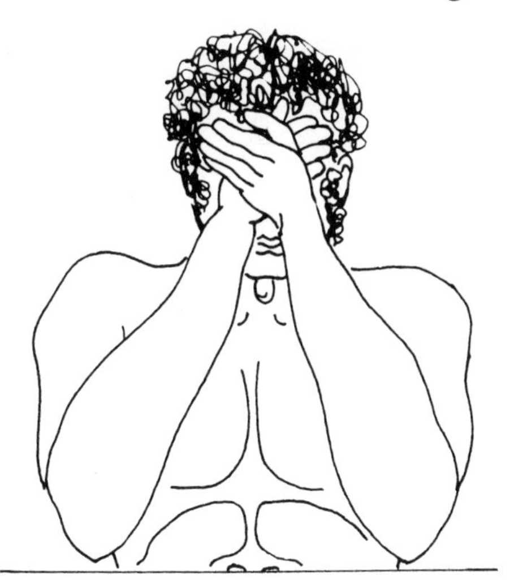

for all people, regardless of their current state of vision. Half a minute when you need it helps; 5 or 10 minutes in the morning and evening is a great idea; even a full hour of continuous palming is not too much. It's the greatest healer of strained eyes-and-mind. Practice it often.

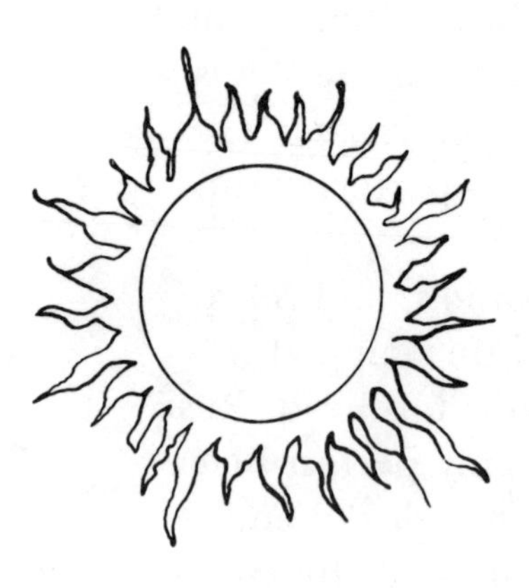

OTHER HEALTH SYSTEMS

I don't mean to make this an encyclopedia of all the existing health systems, but I do want to give you an idea of how many different approaches there are. Here are three more systems whose practices are available to you, if you're interested:

Homeopathic Medicine

This is a complete medical system distinguished by its use of minute dosages of natural drugs obtained from animal, vegetable, and mineral sources. These drugs are used to "charge" the person's own *vital force* into bringing about the healing process. In homeopathic practice each person is treated *uniquely*—the same symptoms may require two completely different treatments for two different people; and as a *whole* entity—that is, the patient's mental and emotional state is considered as well as the physical ailment.

Naturopathy

This is a complete system of health and healing based on natural forces and natural remedies. It includes diet, fasting, internal cleansing, massage of various types, exercises, and the healing properties of the natural elements (air, light, water, heat, electricity)—as well as mental and emotional therapy. Naturopathic physicians are trained in four-year programs at colleges of naturopathic medicine before being licensed to practice. Many of the health techniques mentioned elsewhere in the book are also included in naturopathic practice: breathing exercises, natural-vision training, yogic postures, foot reflexology, air baths, manipulation and massage, natural foods (naturopaths are especially big on living, uncooked foods), natural minerals, mono-diets, food-balancing, and fasting. It is a whole and healthy body-mind system, with one fundamental principle: "Nature cures, not the physician!"

Foot Reflexology

This system is based on the fact that the nerves connecting all the important glands, organs, and parts of the body have terminals (endings) in the feet. Disorders of the body, reflexologists claim, can be alleviated and even permanently cured by pressure and massage at the appropriate points on the feet where these nerve endings are located.

In his natural state man walked barefoot over rough and varied terrain, thus continually massaging his feet and stimulating the nerve reflexes there that connected to the rest of his body. But with our footwear, our smooth floors and streets, and our sedentary indoor lives, this is not the case anymore. Crystalline accumulations build up around the nerve terminals, inhibiting the normal flow of nervous (electrical) energy. Foot reflexology is a way of rubbing off these deposits and stimulating the nerves where required.

You can try this on your own by first massaging all parts of your feet and ankles really well. The places that feel especially sensitive or painful indicate a disorder in the part of your body connecting to the reflex you're pressing in your foot. You should then pay particular attention to those reflexes and massage them gradually but firmly, using your thumbs. Also try to go without shoes as much as you can, and keep your feet in good working condition with plenty of natural movement.

Whatever system you choose to follow, remember that physical inaction is deadly. You were meant to *move!*

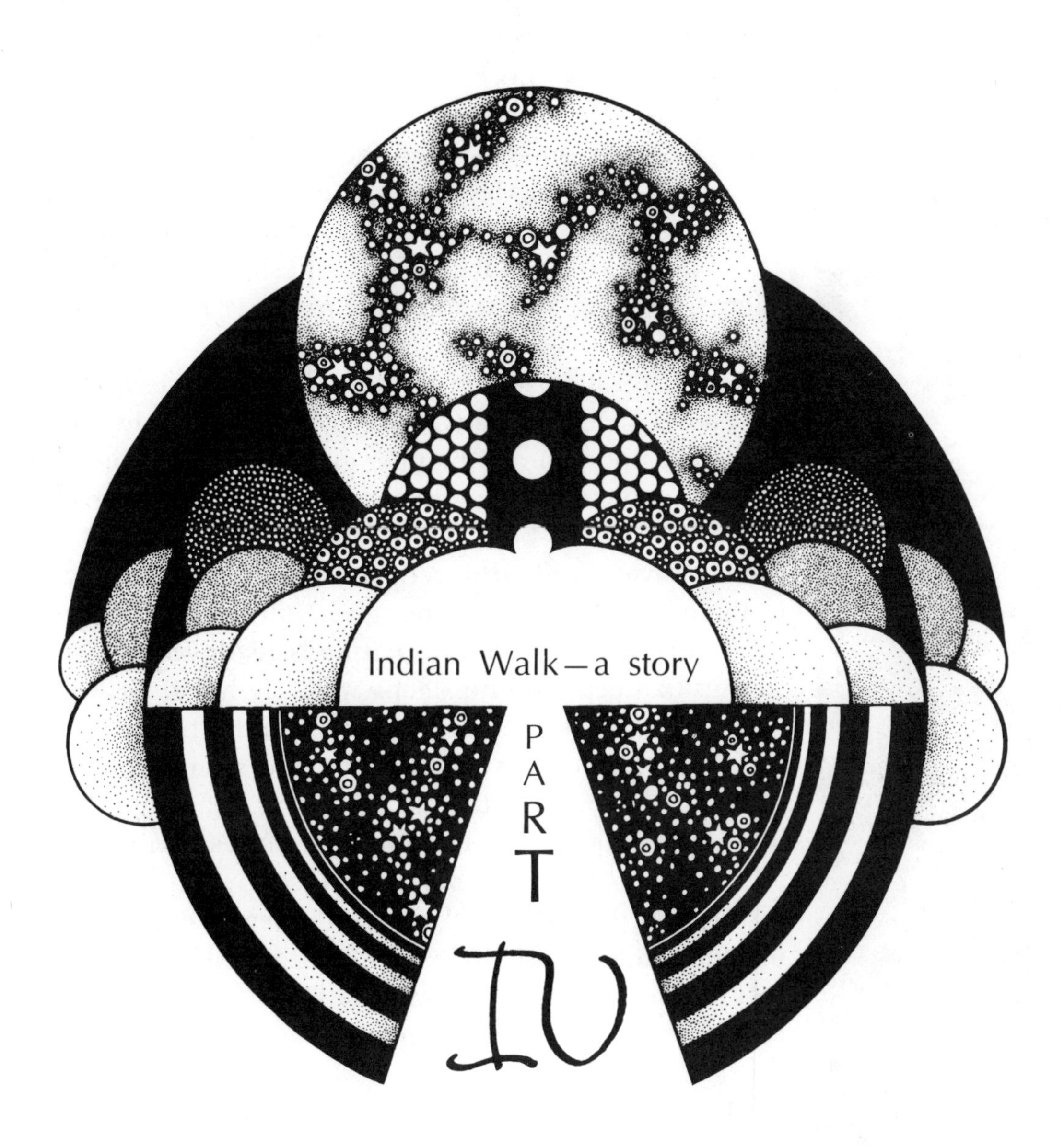
Indian Walk—a story
PART
IV

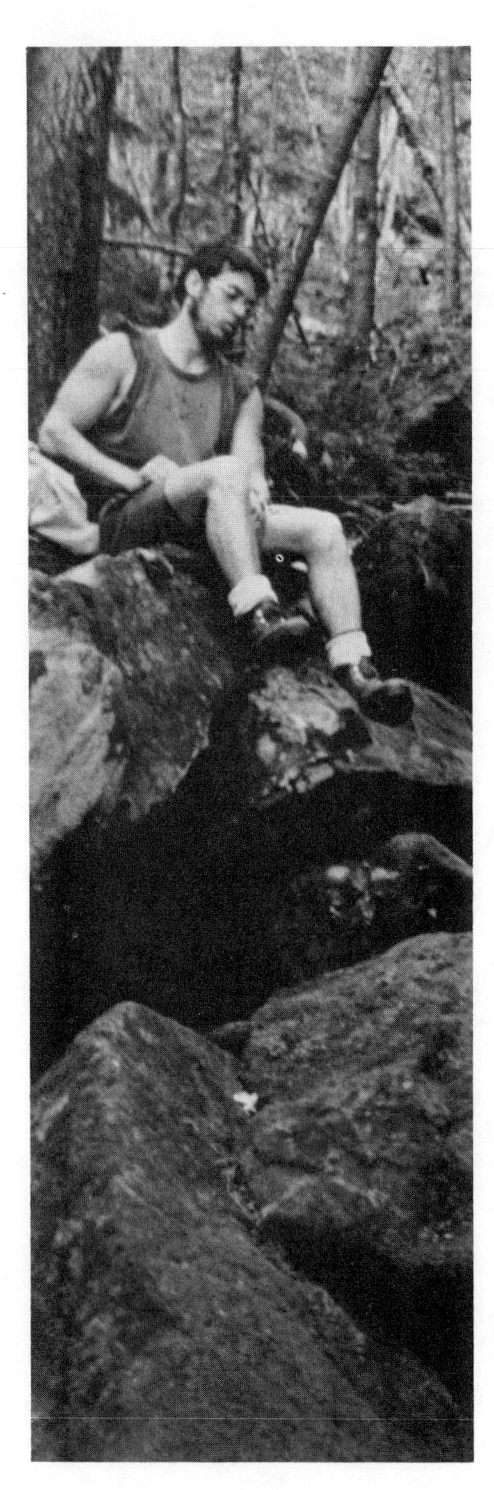

He wakes easily, moving from dream to morning as one goes from one room to another in a familiar house. He lies still for a few moments, keeping his dreams with him as he glides into consciousness and becomes aware of his body. He breathes.

He stretches one leg, then the other; then his arms, neck, back, hips, ankles, until all of him stretches, and his bones crackle. Like a big cat, luxuriating in the sensations of his own well-structured flesh, he feels the energy of being awake and alive reaching every part of him.

He lies on his back on the thin, hard mattress that is his bed. To sleep on this spare pallet that barely softens the wood floor, the body must give itself to gravity and let go completely in the arms of sleep. Not like those soft marshmallow-beds that swallow you up, so that even a tense, rigid, armored, robot body can lie down in them and fall asleep—though it will never sleep well. Therefore he sleeps only when he is ready to give himself up to sleep, and he sleeps well. He has slept well.

He raises his knees until he can feel the full length of his spine from coccyx to skull, flat and straight along the mattress. He breathes in, raises his head slightly and lifts his legs off the bed. Doing this makes him feel his lower belly, where the muscles are contracting to hold his legs up. He kicks and shakes the legs, keeping them up; turns his feet in circles, feeling the ankles; flexes his feet and is aware of their arches. His attention is at his belly. He puts his feet down, lets the air out, opens his eyes.

The room is half-lit with the dawn, just beginning to make colors out of things that have been only degrees of darkness. The room is large, clean, and airy. Through two open windows come the morning breezes, cool with the night's frost but sweet with the opening earth, the buds on tree branches, the wet ground.

He smells the cool and the sweetness, drinking it in with deep, full breaths, filling himself with the morning air. It is late April in the north country. The breeze brings in the sounds of birds and running water. He wants to be in those sounds, in that air, in the morning, without the walls and windowpanes that stand between.

He moves from the center of his body, rising to his feet swiftly and gracefully until he stands, naked, by the window that looks east to where the sky is turning a low shade of orange and a few high clouds are already gold from a sun he cannot yet see. The air is cold moving across his bare skin, which is still warm from sleeping; he puts on a pair of soft, loose corduroy trousers, patched with red and blue bandana cloth. The pants are old and familiar, and fit well; it feels good to put them on.

Then a T-shirt, white, clean, and also soft. A green and black flannel shirt goes on over the T-shirt. He hitches the pants up with a pair of cloth suspenders. He likes the way everything fits—warmly, but without binding or restricting his free movement. Then a pair of wool socks and a pair of tall moccasin-style boots with soft soles, which he has made himself this winter from a deerskin hide. They also fit well—his feet are warm inside them, yet he can feel the ground almost as if he were barefoot. Like the mattress—they soften, but the feeling of contact with the earth remains. He bounces a little in the boots, the pants, the shirt. It all feels right.

He goes out the door, stuffing a red kerchief in his back pocket. Trees are dark against the lightening sky. Air, birds, wind, trees, running water. It will be warm today. But there is still snow, big patches of it in the sloping field across which his morning legs carry him as he heads toward the stream at the far side. Up in the hills the snow is still deep.

He begins running across the field, through a drift,

and feels the grainy softness of the snow. Running into the wind, feeling more of the air as it passes faster through his lungs, smelling more the smells of morning as his breath quickens and deepens with the running.

Nearing the stream, he sees that it is full, moving fast, the snow from the hills melting to make the water sing over the smooth rocks of the stream bed. Without slowing, he angles his run to the left, calculating wordlessly the best place to jump. Reaching the bank, he leaps with a shout, raising his knees high up to his chest to lengthen the jump—and lands, laughing, on two feet, in the snowbank on the opposite side.

He turns and squats, facing the stream. The water calls. He gets a firm footing and kneels over the rushing water. He finds a rock that is close to the shore, puts one hand on it, leans out, lowers his head to the water, and drinks.

The water is cold and fresh. The music of it over the rocks is louder at this closeness. He leans and drinks again, almost losing his handhold on the slippery rock. For fun he pushes off the rock, twists, and quickly switches supporting hands on the wet rock, a split second before he would have fallen face-first into the water. He drinks again, then washes his face with his already wet hand. His eyes love the cool water. He washes forehead, nose, neck, hair. He bends the supporting arm, pushes hard off the rock, and his weight returns to his knees and feet on the earth of the bank. He shakes the water off his hands and squats on his haunches, listening to and looking at the stream.

The cold water has loosened the mucus in his nostrils and sinuses. He takes the kerchief out and clears his nose—first one side, then the other, then both. More air than ever seems to flow into him as he breathes now. He feels the air and it is good.

He turns and continues up the slope, which is steeper now as it rises to the ridge. He turns his long stride into a run again, not wishing to miss the sunrise and feeling a little chilly from the water evaporating off his head. Blood rushes into his thighs as his legs bend deep to pump him up the rise.

He skirts several big drifts of snow without slowing, sees as he runs the pines on one edge of the field, the apple trees on the other; keeps running, snorting to keep his nose clear and to avoid having to breathe in the cold air through his mouth.

The last part of the rise is the steepest and he exhales harder, through his mouth now, to get rid of the used-up air as fast as possible. He sprints straight up the steepest part and reaches the top panting and blowing clouds of mist and pacing like a stallion.

The ridge is a high place. Ahead of him the orange is turning to gold and the clouds are already reflecting the sun's rays, though it is several minutes yet to rising over the spine of the White Mountain range, some thirty miles to the East. He turns around: The West is still dim with the dawn, but he sees his own valley and the house in it, then more hills and the line of the Green Mountains twenty miles off.

The South is all hills, lakes, orchards, brooks, fields, abandoned cabins, secret places that he knows well. The North is dark with clouds and a cold wind blowing down from Canada, through the pine grove, with the distant howl of a winter that has almost finished.

Above him the sky is turning blue; a trace of crescent moon is still visible but giving up its magic to the daylight as each minute passes. Beneath his feet is the earth. Where he stands it is brown, old grasses, old fall leaves of beech, maple, and oak trees—and the thick rich earth soft and wet underneath. No green yet pushes through the brown, but it is ready. A dawn for all things that grow. His body feels tumescent, almost liquid; it feels full not with a ripeness but with the seed-energy of new beginning. Beauty all around—sky, earth, air, water, birds, wind, sunrise. It may be the first day he has ever been alive.

He turns to the East again. A great thing is happening now. He spreads his feet wide apart and bends his knees, lowering himself even closer to the ground. He feels the weight of his attachment to the earth and it is good. Raising his arms, he breathes in slowly, deeply; out slowly, completely. Three times.

On the fourth breath he begins to sing. It just comes out, wells up from his feet, his legs, his belly, and from his heart, announcing his joy at being here on the ridge in April in the North country, with the sun rising.

With every breath he sings, till his lungs empty of air, then fills them and sings again. No person has written this song, and none has heard it but the hills and the raccoons, the jackdaws and the deer in the valley, and now the Sun.

First only a point of light, rays of the brightest gold emanating from that single point; then a small curve that grows, grows, as he still breathes and sings. Then a half-circle of liquid light and everything is changing—the colors, the air, the earth even seems to change beneath his singing feet, and the birds sing also;

now the whole orb appears and he can only look at it in snatches, it seems to hang for a moment by some molten brightness glue to the gold-rimmed mountains, while still he sings; and then it enters the sky, shining miraculously as he has never seen it before; he hears water rushing, wind singing; his own lips close; the day begins.

He lowers his eyes, bends over, covers them with his palms to cool them from the brightness. Rises, turns around, opens them again. Sunlight on things makes long shadows, and warmth. He runs in the direction of his shadow, downhill, with a skipping, leaping, uneven bouncing rhythm. But he feels constrained, kept from letting go and running free and full tilt—by what?

He realizes instantly: by the fear of falling. Only one thing to be done, he knows—plunge into that fear. He makes himself go faster, taking long jolting strides till he is running down the steep decline toward the stream completely without control, heading for the big, sun-flashing-white snowdrift in a hollow of the hill, his fear mounting but also a crazy feeling of indestructibility and joy. It's not clear whether his fall is accidental or deliberate—at the moment it happens there's no time to think about it. Suddenly he loses or gives up his balance and pitches forward, doesn't fight it, goes with it, amplifying the fall with an extra push of his own and tucking his head down, so that he somersaults head over heels, landing on the curve of his back in the soft wet snowdrift with a muffled thud, but he's curved and relaxed so he just keeps rolling down,

and because he rolls and the slope is steep, he is not slowed down, and back on his feet again for only a second, he continues to fall, again adds a push with his legs, bigger this time than the last because the fear left him at that first amazing thud; sails out for a second over the snow, whooping in flight, tucks his head under, lands on his crescent-back again, rolls up to his feet, leaps again, even higher this time, whoops in midair again, tucks, curves, lands, rolls to his feet, continues falling——

notices the approaching trees that line the stream, knows one more roll will bring collision, still no fear but he doesn't leap this time, lets himself fall flat instead, on his front, in the shining snow—a final soft bump. He lies in the snow, laughing.

Then he gets up quickly and shakes the snow from his hands and face. He turns his wet front to the sun, eyes closed; it warms him now. "So much for falling," he says, into the clear air.

Now he follows the path of the stream into the valley, through birch and maple woods, beech woods, magical larch, the little clearings he loves among the young firs, to the lake and the willow tree by it that always is the first to bud, past the old cemetery full of gray gravestones and an apple tree, over rises and through hollows, to other hills, and secret places, by himself but not alone.

And in this way he spends the April morning, walking, trotting, running, crawling; jumping, falling, skipping, climbing trees; kneeling beside streams, singing to the woods, whistling to the birds, breathing. He keeps moving, fast over the open spaces, slower through the thickly forested areas where he has to turn and twist to pass between trees, around bushes, over fallen logs. When he tires he slows down; now and then he lies on his back to look at the sky and a pair of hawks circling high up, on a wind he can only guess at. He passes the morning in a silence of the mind: no plans, no worries, not too many memories. The hours are full, varied, and lively; with trees and brooks and deer, rabbit, squirrels and birds, he lacks not for company. He lets "body" do as he will, lets only instincts and feelings guide him through the woods. He does not think much in the way others are bound up in thinking—not so many words, not so many ideas fill his head. He sees a tree, he does not think "here is a *tree*"; he just sees it, senses it—*feels* it. He listens, he hears; he looks, he sees; he smells, he touches, he tastes; he learns, he knows. No blame. No haste. He laughs.

He sees those things that have died during the winter and will not wake to see this spring; he feels sad for them. He comes upon four huge, tall, white-birch trees that have been downed by some winter storm; their root system lies exposed above the granite it could not cling to. Four brave, strong, straight, tall trees, dying slowly because they could not sink their foundations deep enough into the earth to balance their great upward growth: a forest tragedy. He finds the trees, dying yet still pushing buds forth on their branches; he weeps for them and sings over them. The lesson of the trees.

He climbs and sits beneath an old, gnarled, sturdy maple near the top of a small hill. Small hill, small valley, small stream. The proportions are nice; very understandable.

He sits at the base of the tree with his legs crossed and his back straight. Straight like the four birches. It is warm, the sun shines on his face and hair from its near-noon height; he closes his eyes. He hears life all around. Life, and death too. The birches.

What kind of thing is he? A creature "young" or "old"? Is he being born or dying? Breath comes, heart beats, he is himself—for what purpose? The questions are not thought so much as felt and asked from deep inside him. He sits with these large and real questions, breathing slowly, inheriting some of the old maple tree's slow and consistent nature. It is mid-day.

She got up early today, the first morning of the three-day weekend she had off from work. This holiday came none too soon; for days she'd been staring out the window of the office that overlooked the park, watching the kids playing outside and the ground turning green with the first shoots of new grass, spotted with patches of daffodils. She hated being cooped up in that office.

Certainly, she had *chosen* to live in the city, where her friends, her apartment, and everything familiar to her was. And a young woman on her own couldn't just live anywhere and still have a decent job and make a living for herself. She'd been on this job over a year now, and they liked her there. The pay was all right, enough to live on and save just a little. It was okay. It was okay.

But sometimes she felt that it was not really *her* life that she was living. And only by some effort of will did she accede to the daily necessity of the working-girl clothes, the jostling, noisy ride on the subway every morning and every evening, the long, uninteresting hours at the office. Sitting, that was the worst of it —eight hours of sitting in the same chair, at the same desk—while the green grass was pushing up through the warm earth outside!

Oh yes, she had all the reasons why this life she was leading was the best one for her; but they seemed like reasons for somebody else, reasons that had somehow been mistakenly plugged into *her* body. Her body never did feel right at work; and when she got home, usually it was all she could do to relax a little, watch the news on TV while making a little supper, wash her hair, read a little, clean up, things like that. It wasn't enough of *something!* She'd almost quit smoking—had in fact quit for a while, but started again when things got sort of tense at work. Now she only smoked a few a day; that was okay. . . . She'd bought a book on Yoga and relaxation and tried to spend half an hour or so almost every day doing the breathing exercises and practicing the postures. This seemed to help, especially after work; it made her feel more peaceful and content with herself. But why did it have to be that way, why should she have to *practice* relaxing? Why wasn't she able to just feel good with herself *all* the time? And what was she doing at that stupid job anyway? She had always thought her life was going to amount to something—but this sure wasn't it!

Thoughts and feelings like this had been bothering her for a long time now, but there didn't seem to be anyone she could talk to about them. Then came the letter, from the guy she'd met on that freezing day in February. (They'd both been out walking by the Charles River, no one else in sight, the wind was blowing like mad and then it started to snow really heavy, and there was so much space and air and everything was beautiful

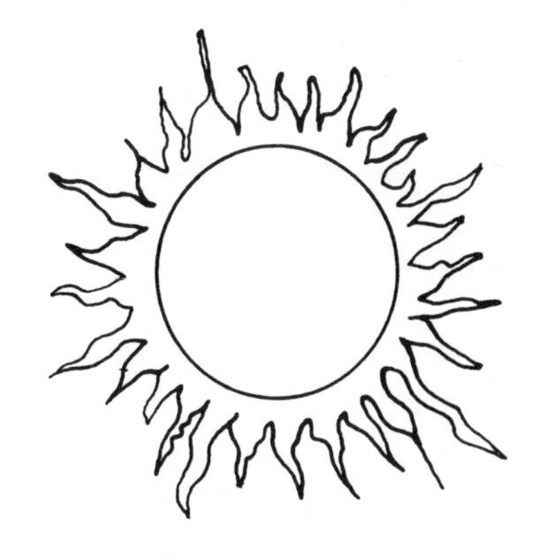

in the snow, and there was this guy, just kind of walking around, with his coat open and no hat on, and he put his head back to look up at the snow and let it fall on his face, and he looked *happy,* like nobody she'd seen in a long time, and she put her head back and let the snow fall on her face too, and she started laughing and he noticed and they laughed together, and then they walked along by the river for a while in this terrific snowstorm without talking a whole lot but they just looked at each other and played funny sorts of games, like kids do, and she really felt happy too, and alive, and then they went and had some coffee and talked for quite a while but she didn't remember too much of exactly what they talked about, except that he lived in an old house up in Vermont, and he told her that because they laughed together that was an important thing and how when the Eskimos make love they call it "laughing together," that's their way of saying it, and she remembered that his hands looked like good hands and that he didn't look away when she looked straight into his eyes. And that was all on a Sunday afternoon and she went back to work the next day although she couldn't really see the point.) And his letter was an invitation to come up and spend the three days with him at his place in some remote part of Vermont, and it was simply written but clear and strong and happy. It made her remember that time in the snowstorm. She had written him back immediately, saying yes.

She stood drying herself in front of the full-length mirror in her bedroom, after a nice hot morning shower. She saw a naked young woman, not unattractive, in reasonably good health and neither too fat nor too thin. A kind face, sensitive eyes—but who *was* this person facing her? She could not determine the feelings of the young woman in the mirror, and it began to scare her a little, so she quickly turned away and put on her usual weekend clothes. She was anxious to get away—and to see what this strange man who sent her the letter was really like!

She closed her bags, locked the double locks on her apartment door, walked downstairs, checked the mailbox, put the bags in the car, got in, started the engine. She noticed that it was a nice day. The engine made a lot of noise on the otherwise quiet residential street. While the engine warmed up she checked the tires, then looked over at where the sun had just appeared over a row of buildings and the sky was all orange and gold above the line of old brick houses. She got back in the car, locked the door, put on her seat belt, put a pack of cigarettes on the dashboard, and drove off.

It was earlier than the hour she went to work. The city looked different, as if the mask of its workday identity had been taken off during the night and not yet replaced. She remembered it was a holiday, and it pleased her to think that everything might stay looking like this for the whole day.

She saw things she'd never noticed before: the jagged line of rooftops, the square corners of the buildings and the streets, the city colors—concrete gray, brick brown, asphalt black. She saw the city naked in its architecture, its square unbreathing forms; and beneath the structures she could discern the shape of a land that once rolled gently in greens and browns down to the waters that once were only blue. So this is all the earth too, only with us on top of it, she thought as she headed up the ramp onto the superhighway going north.

The drive wasn't more than an hour old when she began to feel uncomfortable. Her legs had no energy, her buttocks were immobilized, her pelvis and groin deadened. Her shoulders were beginning to tighten up, and she was feeling the strain behind and around her eyes. She also noticed that her breathing was shallow, irregular—just the opposite of the Yoga breathing she'd been practicing. And she was smoking entirely too much. She pulled off the road at the next opportunity into the highway service area.

When she turned the engine off she realized how much its steady drone had permeated her senses. It took her hearing a full minute to get back to normal. She got out of the car and locked it. She tried to loosen up her tight muscles by stretching, bending, and twisting her body around; her spine cracked loudly with each twist. But her shoulders were still tight, her legs numb. So she started to bounce on her toes, letting her arms dangle loosely from their sockets. That made her legs begin to come alive, and relaxed her shoulders some. She closed her eyes to give them a rest, while she kept on bouncing. It felt good to be moving her body. She hummed a little tune to herself and just let the air go in and out of her in long, deep breaths.

Then it occurred to her: what if people see me doing this, a grown person jumping up and down and humming with her eyes closed in a service area parking lot—they'll think I'm crazy for sure; and she stopped. With a little sigh she turned and walked into the restaurant.

The "restaurant" was a row of shiny plastic vending machines. She looked carefully at all the machines—soft drinks, candy, chocolate, cigarettes, plastic-wrapped sandwiches on white bread. None of it looked like what she needed. But she needed *something.* She put a dime and a nickel in the Hot Drinks machine and pressed the button for "Coffee—Light, no Sugar." Out it came, not very hot, not tasting very much like coffee. She drank from the paper cup while reading the headlines on the newspapers encased in a plastic vendor. All the headlines were about violence somewhere—or money, it seemed to her. Or else about politics, which was just some combination of the two. She couldn't finish the coffee, and threw the half-full cup into the plastic garbage receptacle near the glass doors that led out of the restaurant. It occurred to her that spilling the liquid into the garbage can would make the job of emptying the can only that much more unpleasant for the poor man whose means of living it was to empty those cans—but what should she have done with it instead? It occurred to her that she might have emptied it down the sink in the ladies' room; but the thought came too late, she'd already dropped the cup into the garbage.

Not much of a rest stop, she smiled ironically to herself. She filled up the car with gas. The exhaust fumes of the other cars idling their engines while being tanked up seemed to choke her so that she hardly wanted to breathe. The service station attendant glared at her when she asked him to clean the windshield. There was nothing to be done about it all. She paid for the gas and drove on.

Gradually, seen through the thick glass of windshield and windows, the urban sprawl gave way to countryside. There were more trees and fewer houses; more open fields, more space, fewer factories and smokestacks. Neon signs and polluted air were slowly being transformed, as she drove, into weathered barns, evergreen trees, and clear sunlight.

She opened the windows of the car; the air was better. She breathed in, deeply—and smiled. The towns the highway passed were becoming fewer and smaller and farther apart. Here and there the road afforded views of mountains still white-capped, rolling hills descending to fertile valleys beribboned with rivers. The sun was shining. She felt better. With effort she concentrated on the road and her driving. But it wasn't so unpleasant now, being surrounded by so much beauty.

After another hour of driving she exited off the highway. Then more driving, along a two-lane blacktop road that passed through smaller towns, curved and wound around hills, over smaller rivers, past old farmhouses. The uncomfortableness of the driving increased, her hips and legs were feeling dead again, her eyes had grown tired of staring at the road. But she was excited to be in the country, and the discomfort could be endured for that.

Coming around a long curve at the base of a steep hill, she saw, up and off the road to the right, a waterfall! She pulled the car off to the side, turned the motor off, and got out. She walked a few yards into the snow by the side of the road and stood there, looking and listening. The sound of the waterfall was all she heard. She saw *water falling;* she had never seen such a thing before! It cascaded downward in three long graceful leaps, from stream bed, over cliff and through air, onto rock, off rock and into air, and became stream-water again. She let the sound and beauty of the fall fill her for a long moment, then walked back to the car.

The last few miles were along a narrow dirt road that led up and away from the blacktop. There were no houses to be seen along that road, only woods and fields. The road was muddy. She drove slowly, in low gear to maintain traction in the mud; she learned the land a little going so slowly, and she felt less separated from it.

Coming over a rise after several miles of this slow muddriving, she saw the house. It was set at the upper end of a long valley, the full extent of which was lost in the distance. A sloping field led from the house to a steep ridge, then seemed to fall away; the next visible thing in that direction was a line of mountains, white-peaked and far off.

The house is old, gray-shingled, weathered; she can see a woodpile standing to the valley side of it. She stops the car and turns off the engine. She is already smiling. . . .

She gets out of the car. The quietness immediately washes her, a quietness that is not silence. Slowly, sounds sort themselves out: water rushing, birds calling, wind blowing through evergreens.

She walks around the house once, seeing lake, stream, field, ridge, valley, mountains. Sees the woodpile, neat stacks of thick logs, the shorter cylinders of logs that have been sawed, stacks of quarter-splits from these cylinders, a chopping block, a sawhorse. Efficient, and beautiful. There is a garden plot, the ground already turned, and the dark, wet, fertile brown soil exposed; it smells good to her. A compost pile at the farther end of the plot. Good, good. She completes the circuit around the house and comes to the front again. She sees her own car, thinks about locking the doors, and smiles—no need to lock them. The midday sun shines on her standing there.

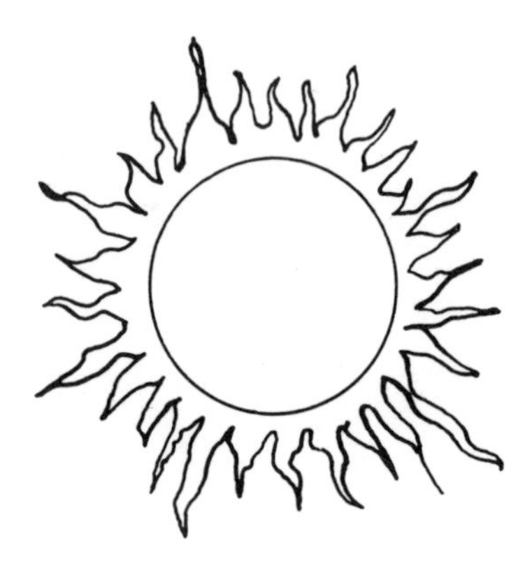

He had been sitting under the maple tree until his mind quieted, until brain and spine ceased to be at odds and he could know why he moved and lived. It came from below first, the Call, like some surplus of energy that stirred in him, beyond the cycles he had already acknowledged and balanced within himself—breathing, eating, sleeping, heart beating. This was something more, it made him feel, whole as he was, the need to move, for a certain energy to be released and used.

He felt it especially at two of the Seven Centers—the genitals and the heart. It was there through no effort of his own, and through no effort could he deny it. He thought of her, the girl in the snow by the river, the laughing, his letter, her reply, her coming today. He knew then that she was there, and smiled . . .

He rises, stretches and shakes his body, like a mountain lion after a long sleep on a high rock. Walks, with long strides, down from the maple tree toward the house, singing. His blood moves well inside him, and his head is clear and light upon his shoulders. He feels the earth under his broad feet. He walks to her.

She is in the house, in his room, seeing the way his things are kept, seeing the mattress low on the floor and the candle beside it; seeing the desk and the kerosene lamp that stands on it; the bookshelf made from barnboards and bricks, and the books in it; seeing the many things made of wood, the dried wildflowers in vases, herbs in bunches hung behind doors, pictures on the walls—the poetry and life of his room. She is in the room, feeling right about being there. Such a freeing, yet ordered place! She feels relieved here, and relaxed —but also excited in a way. She feels womanly.

Through the open window she hears a voice coming from the hillside across the valley, a man's voice. Sun streams in the window, the wind plays, and there are other sounds, but it is only the voice that she hears. She slips off her coat and leaves it in the room. She goes outside. It's sunny.

A path leads down from the house, then up the other side of the valley, where the voice comes from. She begins walking that way, and the city fades from her with every step. She breathes, she walks. Her hips sway and she begins to sing also, so he will know her coming. The ground is soft. Buds appearing on the trees. Air is alive. Singing, they see each other.

May their roads home be on the trail of peace
Happily may they all return

In beauty I walk
With beauty before me I walk
With beauty behind me I walk
With beauty above me I walk
With beauty around me I walk
In beauty it is finished
In beauty it is finished

NAVAHO

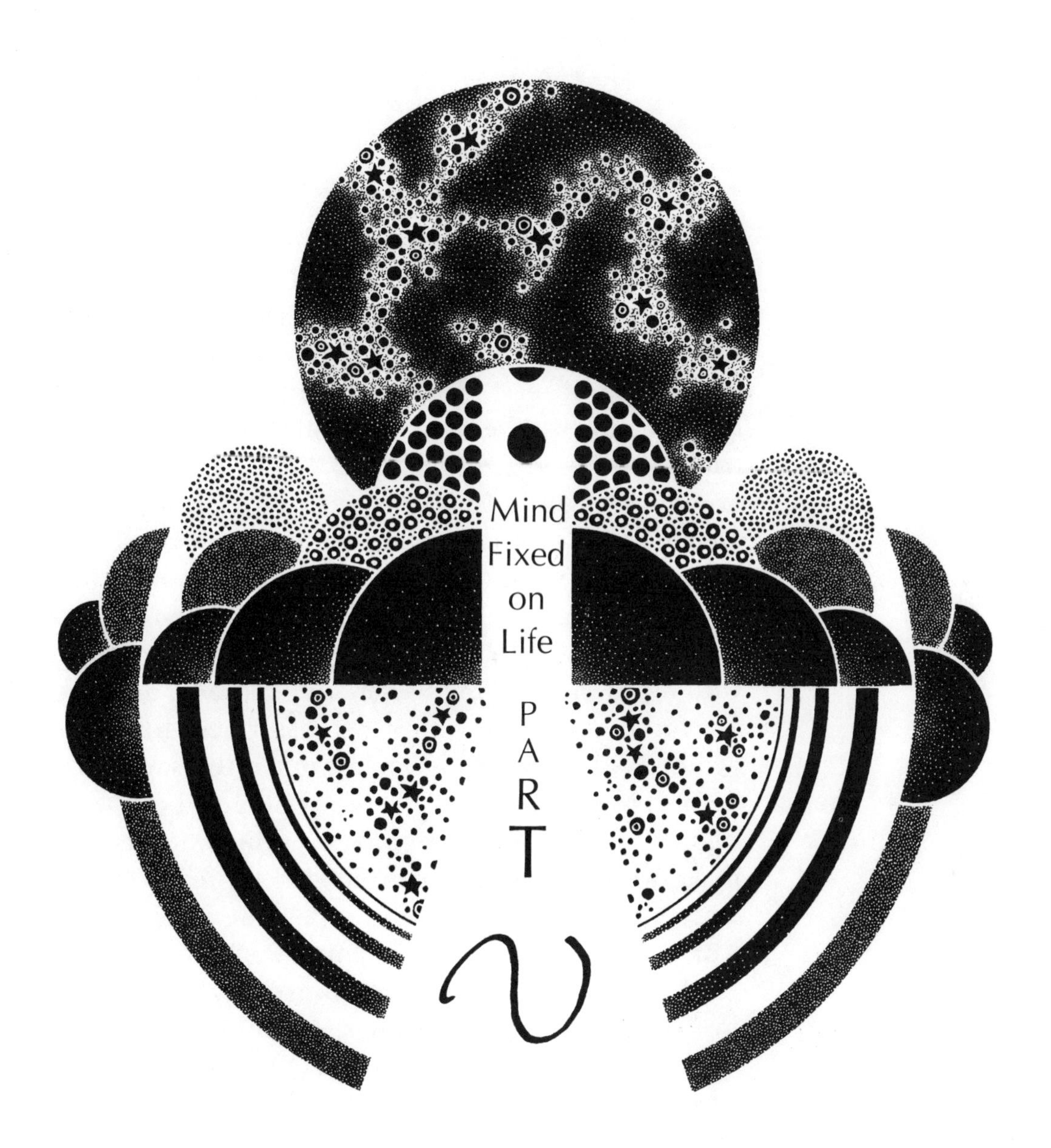
Mind
Fixed
on
Life
PART
V

THE FORM

Separation-Initiation-Return: The hero, or heroine, departs from the everyday world of society, habit, role-playing, and commonplace sufferings. An adventure is undertaken that leads into strange lands and includes the encountering of mysterious and dangerous forces. Though the journey may be a physical one, and the trials met be trials of the body, ultimately the difficulties encountered are known also to be forms of the dark forces within the adventurer's own character, within the unconscious. Finally a kind of victory is won; a certain coming to terms with the cosmos, a union with the unknown, a reconciliation with all that was feared. The seeker is filled with a power, a divine life-energy, a grace, a transcendent force. And then returns, transformed, to the world again; lives outwardly perhaps, much the same as before; but is changed, is new, is able to bestow the boon of his or her own grace on others, to heal, to make whole what has been divided, to make peace where there was war, to bring new life into the dark world, and (if only in some small way) to redeem it.

This pattern we encounter constantly. If one day you just go out and walk 10 miles, or run for an hour, or keep perfect silence for a whole morning, you will see what I mean. You will enter another reality, you will deal with forces and problems unlike those of everyday life; at some point the greatest difficulty will be overcome, and you will feel a change. And when you return, finally, you will have gained some small but definite particle of power, or grace, or ch'i, or new life-energy. The names are not important. Just try it.

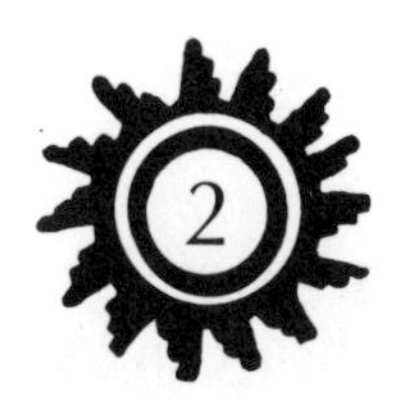

THE FEET

Feet are your contact points with the earth. Physically they form the opposite pole from the head. In the East they say "cool head-warm feet" is a sign of health and a balanced personality. If your feet are strong this is a firm, balanced base from which the rest of you can be well-supported. (If your feet are weak or not used naturally, many problems can arise. For example, weak arches do not cushion the shocks of walking, running, jumping as well as strong arches; this shock may then be felt elsewhere, even at the brain. Headaches and even more serious disorders can result. Improper foot structure or position while standing or walking can cause the pelvis to tilt forward or backward from the vertical, putting pressure on the lower spinal vertebrae, which in turn can produce pain and various disorders of the nervous system.)

Pay attention to your feet. Go barefoot when you can, especially out of doors on natural surfaces like grass, earth, sand, and rock. Massage your feet regularly, make them more sensitive, more "conscious." Exchanging sensuous foot massages with someone you love is a beautiful thing. Feet are the least respected, least attended to parts of the anatomy; when someone lavishes care and attention on your heels, your middle toes, your arches, your ankles, you feel—very well-loved, to say the least.

And shoes. Shoes can be very destructive weapons to your health and well-being! Good shoes leave your feet free rather than constricted, let them breathe rather than sweat and suffocate, soften the hardness or rough-

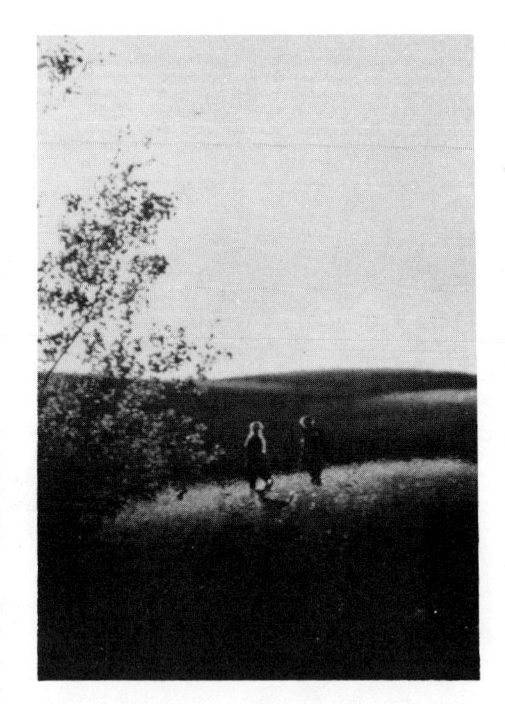

ness of the surfaces you walk on without breaking or distorting your sense of contact with the earth. Regardless of the fashion, the only good shoe is one that *feels* good to walk in.

Walking. Walking is beautiful. Don't take it for granted! Try walking for a solid hour, or a whole morning, without once stopping or breaking your stride. You learn a lot by walking. Feel your feet as you walk. Keep them straight ahead, not splayed out or toed in. Feel your walk change on different surfaces. Walk everywhere you can. Everyone who knows anything about health will agree with this: Don't ride in cars, elevators, golfcarts, motorcycles, buses, subways—*walk!*

Living in your feet, walking a lot, going barefoot or wearing comfortable footwear—these all serve to intensify your feeling of closeness to the earth, of centeredness in your abdomen, of positive energy coming up from your feet and legs through the hips and waist. A very good, strong, balanced feeling. Probably the greatest enemy of this feeling is sitting in chairs. Chairs are death to the lower body! How many hours a day do you sit? Is it absolutely necessary? Try going a whole day without sitting down once: Stand, or kneel, or squat, or lie down, but don't sit on your ass! See how this makes you feel. At this time I'm not going to go into all the reasons why too much chair-sitting is unhealthy; if you're sensitive to your body you can feel it yourself. And if you feel it, then probably you realize how many hours a day you sit. Then you can begin to change your habits.

If your feet, ankles, or calves are weak, invent exercises to strengthen them. If they are inflexible (which is almost always the case with a weak part of the anatomy, for flexibility and strength go together!), invent exercises to loosen them. Your feet are your foundations!

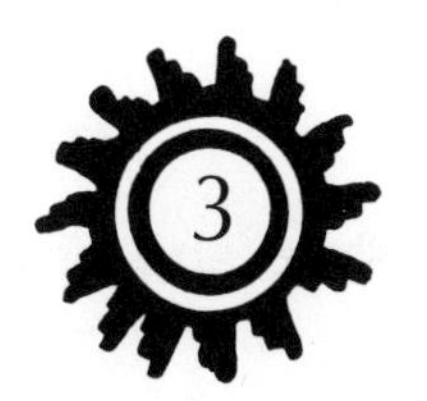

REST

Most of us don't know how to rest. There are many different ways: Running may be a rest—from the strain of physical inactivity, or mental overactivity. Sleep may *not* be a rest, if you go to sleep tense, or upset, or force yourself to sleep with pills. Fasting for a few days is a rest for your digestive system. Palming is a rest, humor is a rest, rhythm is a rest.

Meditation is a rest for the conscious mind. Sleep is also mainly for the mind. (Your *body* is capable of far greater endurance and energy expenditure than you could imagine, without serious fatigue; and it is able to rest and recuperate very easily by any of a number of other relaxation methods, which are at least as good as sleep for this purpose.) In sleep, the conscious mind gives up its tight hold on the reins of your existence, and the forces of the unconscious express themselves.

Yoga masters, who seem to have achieved the integration of the conscious mind with certain areas of (what is still to most of us) the unconscious, are said to do quite well on one or two hours of sleep a night; and some, it is said, need no sleep at all. They get all the mental rest they need from meditation—and the body, as I said, is not dependent on sleep for its survival. This perhaps farfetched-sounding claim about the Yogis is corroborated by a recent finding that a certain Yogin, being tested on a brain-wave measuring machine, was able *at will* to produce the brain waves of both the dreaming state and of the deepest, dreamless sleep—while he remained awake and fully conscious! (Let *that* one be a lesson to you.)

The Passive Relaxation position described earlier is a good rest. Massage can be a delightful rest. Palming is an excellent and much-needed rest for the eyes—like meditation, it can be a descent into the darkness of the sleep state, yet done while you are fully awake. In a way, all spontaneous, unplanned, natural activity and expression of feeling is a rest for us repressed, over-civilized animals. Yell when you feel like it, weep when you feel like it, break a plate when you feel like it—you need the rest!

A Zen master, asked what was the secret of his enlightenment, replied, "Eat when hungry. Sleep when tired." Yes.

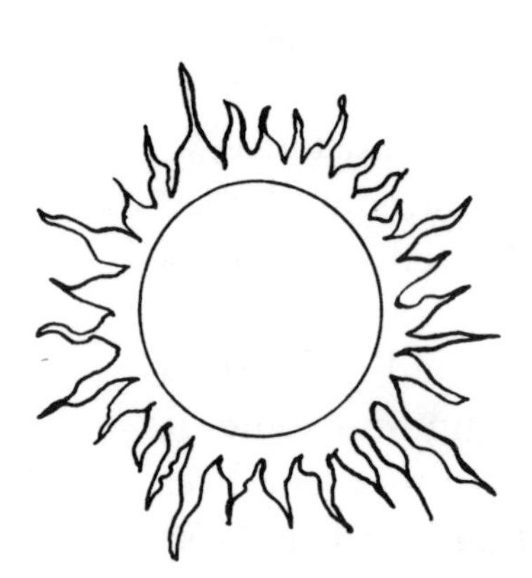

SOME OF MY TEACHERS SPEAK

You have noticed that the truth comes into this world with two faces. One is sad with suffering, and the other laughs; but it is the same face, laughing or weeping. When people are already in despair, maybe the laughing face is better for them; and when they feel too good and are too sure of being safe, maybe the weeping face is better for them to see.

BLACK ELK

When crowds assemble in Trafalgar Square to cheer to the echo the announcement that the government has decided to have them all killed, they would not do so if they had all walked 25 miles that day.

BERTRAND RUSSELL

God is Life.

WILHELM REICH

To reconcile body and spirit would be to recover the breath-soul which is the life-soul instead of the ghost-soul or shadow; breath-consciousness instead of brain-consciousness; body-consciousness instead of head-consciousness. The word made flesh is a living word, not a scripture but a breathing. A line that comes from the breath, from the heart by way of the breath. Aphorism as utterance: a short breath, drawn in pain. Winged words, birds released from the sentence, doves of the spirit.

NORMAN O. BROWN

SWEAT

A T'ai Chi master told me this story:

There was a gathering of all the oldest men in the province, limited to those who had passed the 70-year mark and including a number of spry old fellows in their 80s and 90s, if not older. They were trying to determine the secret of their collective longevity. One after another, they explained their various diets, exercise systems, herbal medicines, special ways of living; but they could come to no general agreement about any of these things. Finally they realized the one element they all had in common was that each managed, in one way or another, to make himself *sweat every day.* And this was their secret.

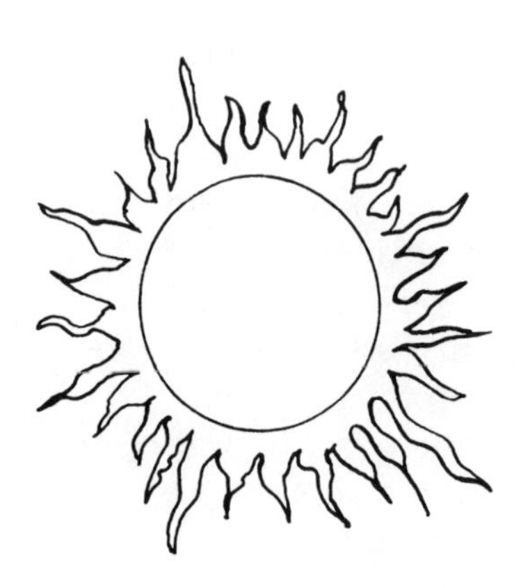

BOOKS

Ellsworth Baker, *Man in the Trap*

W. H. Bates, *Better Eyesight Without Glasses*

Joseph Campbell, *The Hero with a Thousand Faces*

Cheng Man-Ch'ing, *T'ai Chi*

Kenneth Cooper, *Aerobics*

Margaret Darst Corbett, *Help Yourself to Better Sight*

Indra Devi, *Yoga for Americans*

Aldous Huxley, *The Art of Seeing*

Nikos Kazantzakis, *Zorba the Greek*

————, *The Saviors of God*

Alexander Lowen, *Love and Orgasm*

————, *Pleasure*

John G. Niehardt, *Black Elk Speaks*

Wilhelm Reich, *The Function of the Orgasm*

————, *The Murder of Christ*

Koichi Tohei, *Aikido in Daily Life*

Lao Tzu, *Tao Te Ching*

Adele Westbrook and Oscar Ratti, *Aikido and the Dynamic Sphere*

Selvarajan Yesudian and Elisabeth Haich, *Yoga and Health*

FOUR STEPS

A sweltering hot August afternoon, near the end of a two-hour Korean Karate class held in a small upstairs room of a college gym. We are kneeling in the Zen posture; sweat pours from our faces onto the hardwood floor. The teacher, Jin Woong Kim, is speaking. He moves as he talks, but never displaying more than a tiny fraction of the vast energies he has at his disposal. I have seen him kill flies in midflight with a single lightning stroke of his hand-edge, so they were dead before they hit the ground. His ability to kick is terrifying. He is also a very mild person, to the point of shyness.

He is speaking about something he knows—the taking on of a discipline as a way of self-development. The furthest reaches of his art, Karate, are the infinite possibilities of the human system. He says four words, and repeats them:

ACTION

ACTUALITY

FREEDOM

DAILY LIFE

We remember them, and only later understand what he means: It starts in action, movement, the exercise of energy, the practice of *doing.* In the case of Karate, this means learning how to execute kicks, blocks, and strikes in the most efficient and powerful manner.

Then, actuality, which means dealing with circumstances and forces outside yourself. Becoming more *aware* of what is going on, on all levels. Sharpening the senses, honing the reflexes, seeing clearly what *is.* In Karate this means *response*—how to defend against an attack. These first two stages are essentially technical, and can be achieved more or less easily.

The third stage, freedom, means to be neither attacker nor defender, neither compelled by your own imbalances nor ruled by imbalances of others. Bound by nothing, controlled by nothing—but free to live and free to choose. This is no longer a matter of technique but an attitude, a way of traveling.

Finally, daily life. This is the Return I spoke of earlier. What use are freedom, action, actuality—if not in daily life? What good are power, wisdom, personal development—if not to better the world in some way, and to aid all living things?

Having taken the long and painful path of training himself, the martial artist, the wanderer, the sufferer of many defeats and many losses, rounds another curve in the road of his life, to find himself where he began. The daily life of man and woman—the miracles of sleeping, waking, seeing, working, feeling, cooking, making love, being children and having children, eating, drinking, laughing—to live these well is the highest attainment.

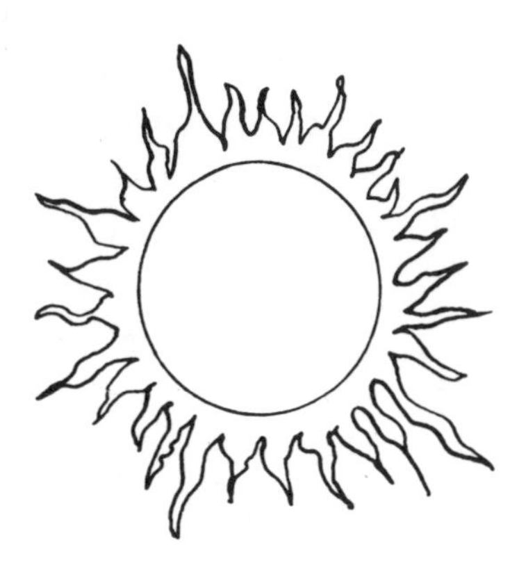

A NOTE

In the Bates Eye System there is a quality of the healthy perfectly-seeing eye called Central Fixation. This means that the eye sees most clearly the one point directly looked at—and less clearly all areas as they recede from that central point. In the abnormal, deficient-vision eye, Central Fixation is always absent or distorted. Bates found that if a person with poor vision could acquire perfect Central Fixation, then his natural, perfect vision would be restored.

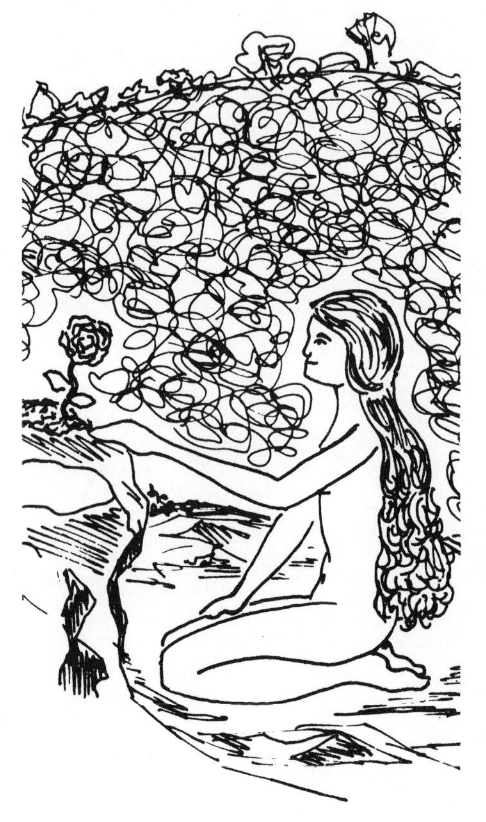

However, as a method of reacquiring this ability, having the patient try to see the central point *more* clearly than the surrounding areas was not only hopeless (if he could *make* himself see better he would have done so long before!) but it actually made his vision worse, from the straining to see. Instead, Bates had his patients imagine that they were seeing all areas away from the center *less well* than the central point. In this way the mind-and-eye of the patient relaxed, and naturally focused itself on the center.

This is a good analogy for living. The conscious mind serves best not by *trying* to do anything but by helping to remove obstacles to a natural unfolding of the real self. (Don't try so hard to do it right—relax and give up doing it wrong!)

My whole message has been: Find your own balance. Don't bother following anyone else. Live as you want to live. All you need is a little bravery, and a lot of love. Get your mind fixed on living, brothers and sisters—that's the secret. Try it and see.

PARTING

I've said enough. Guides only take you part of the way. You go on from here. It's been nice traveling with you.

Be well.

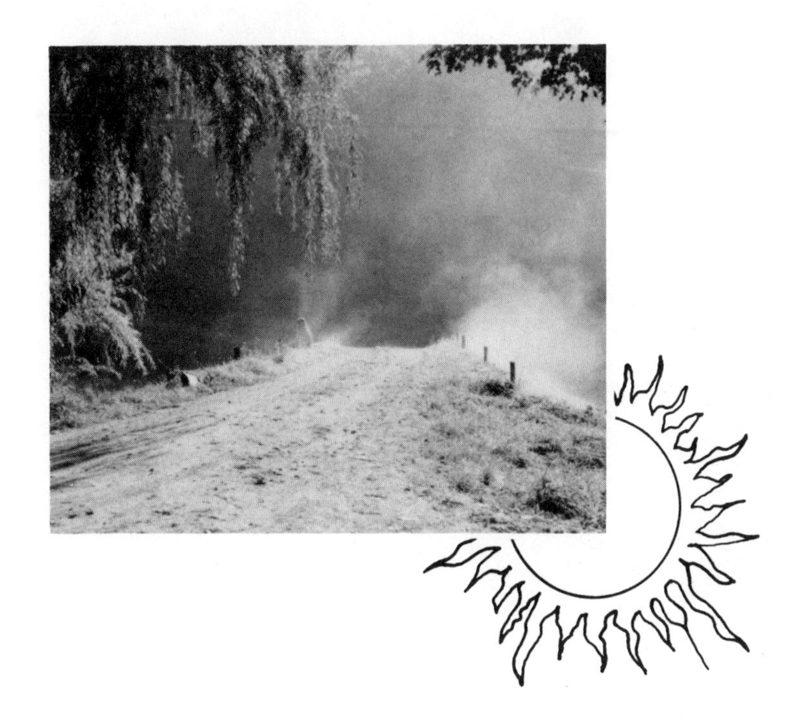